CAUSES OF VARIOUS PHYSICAL AND SPIRITUAL DISEASES

Causes Of Various Physical And Spiritual Diseases

Author's Name

Didik Mulyadi

Editors' Names

Rio Hermawan
Wendy Mulyadi
Ronald Djumani

Cover Design

Rio Hermawan

Bayu Aji Publisher
2016

First Printing: 2016

ISBN 978-1-365-06985-7

Bayu Aji Publisher
Mawar Street 47
Malang, Indonesia, 65154

www.hivaids-medic.com

Contents

Foreword

To all of readers to whom we respect and glorified by God the Almighty wherever you are. We want to give a little advice, if reading on religious things, so the way to read must be repeated, then your heart will be open and more sensitive to differ which is correct and which is wrong.

For you reading the disease causes, this writing is for all humans in all nations as well as all religions. Thus our regard.

Writer

Didik Mulyadi

Chapter 1: Disease Cause

Disease Causes

Disease causes are not food or heredity. They are from ourselves behavior and attitude. The following will be discussed on some disease causes and the ways to prevent.

1. Cause of Hypertension

Cause of hypertension for a Moslem is that he conducts the obligatory worships by being lazy if he conducts sunnah worships by great spirit (oblige the sunnah and making the sunnah as obligation). While for non-Moslems, if facing a big problem, they underestimate it but if facing small problem, they exaggerate it. In this world, there is no result without a cause and there is no cause with no result. The behavior above is not because one has big motivation to worship but because of big reward for the worships. If this behavior is not corrected immediately so one will be easily get hypertension or stroke.

My brothers, prioritize the main things, I believe you will be healthy spiritually and physically. What mean by the main things is the obligatory by God the Almighty namely the *syariah* (two sentences of confession of faith; prayers; alm; fasting in holy month of Ramadhan because of Allah SWT and not because of reward; and pilgrim to Mecca if being able). If the obligations are conducted in a whole because of Allah SWT then undoubtedly that all sunnahs will be sincere and if praying for someone, this will be sincere. Being sincere has the similar value to the obligations namely worships.

Based on the purpose that Allah SWT created human beings in the world, there are many sincere persons, do not want corruption, and being honest; but the problem is not because of corruption but because of being fear of Allah SWT, but because of being fear to be caught or known by others. If the obligations are conducted correctly and because of Allah SWT, so avoiding the His prohibitions is not because of being fear to be caught but because of fear of Allah SWT. It is called as faith.

2. Cause of Diseases in Heart, Breasts, and Cervical Cancer.

For you with diseases in heart, breasts and cervical cancer, you should maintain your heart from any prejudice toward your spouse. One prefers to give prayers because of women so, he will be lose his way then he will also get suffered for a longer time because of women. This is the similar way as worshipping women by Islam way.

The way to heal heart disease is by doing treatment and maintaining the relationship with spouse. Clean the prejudice toward spouse. Indeed, the spouse badness is our reflection because the spouse behavior is the heart reflection. Thus, change your heart by confessing that all of the goods are from

Allah SWT and the bad things are from ourselves, that is called as 'ourselves'. At health condition and never prejudice toward the spouse, so one may not get any heart disease.

Human beings are the most invisible creature; in human body, there are many various types of invisible things. The invisible things in human body are from the core of land for main demand such as eating, the invisible things from the core of fire for main demand of marrying, the invisible things from the core of water for the main demand to drink, and the invisible things from the core of wind for the main demand to breath, the four are called as anger. Also, there is an invisible thing from the core of month for the main demand for sleep, it is called as *alumuah* and the invisible thing from the core of sun is for the main demand for staying awake and it is called as *sufia*. There is also an invisible thing called as *mutmainnah* as the visible things for the main demand to worship because of Allah SWT.

All explanations above are the main demands while there are a lot more other desires. But, the most dominant one controlling this body is the heart having correlation to the visible thing from fire namely to marry / relationship with spouse. Thus, undoubtedly there is a correlation between spouses so, just do good to your spouse, indeed there will be no any disorder to the heart.

All disasters in this world are from the four invisible things above, namely land, fire, water and wind because devils control the invisible things from the seven surface to earth. The four invisible things explained previously are called as body (anger). The invisible thing from land has correlation to the lung, the invisible thing from fire has correlation to the heart, the invisible thing from water has correlation to the pancreas, and the invisible thing from wind has correlation to the liver / bile. The cause of disease has correlation directly to one's behavior and attitude. All prohibitions in Holy Quran can affect negatively on body. The genie who has a throne in the middle of the sun is the Ifrit. Ifrit is a genie confronting the Prophet Muhammad at the time of Ascension. Ifrit's men confront someone who pray for Allah becomes of heaven worship, because of *Intercessory*, and worship because of reward. Therefore whatever happens, just remain worship only for Allah. *Allah says none can intercede with Allah SWT without his permission* (QS. Al-Baqqrah: 255).

Precisely, in the middle of month, there is a genie throne, the woman genie is named as Balqis. At the time of the Prophet Sulaiman AS, the genie scared people into worship for fear of hell. Someone who worships as hell means he is being deceived. Has hell does not exist then the person is guaranteed not to worship. We are also afraid of hell but we were afraid to God in terms of His bans. Someone worshiping for fear of hell is usually jumpy, easy to complain, always anxious, weepy, and precisely does not accept the provisions of Allah SWT. The person does not make Islam as his faith but as doubts and always prejudiced by anyone. When worshiping for Allah then the person has a belief and any measures being undertaken there will be no doubt. Worshiper because Allah will always get the guidance and protection of Allah SWT and their extended family to the *day of apocalypse.*

Worship for heaven can make a person feel to be the most correct person and most sacred feel so, assuming everyone else is dirty. The reason is the creature from the sun controlling so that it makes the feeling to be able to illuminate the whole universe. In fact, only half of the earth is bright. Those are the people who are deceived and lose money in the world and the hereafter. The light of Prophet can only penetrate across the darkness. We also personally request to God in the prayers (obligatory).

3. Causes of Stroke

The cause of stroke is the characteristic to admit a kindness. Surely none goodness is except by His will (the goods are from Allah SWT and the bad is from the man himself). Do not have the characteristic of envy regarding fortune, marriage, and death / birth because they are already determined by God before man was born. For the amount of income, your partner now, and the number of children you have then give thanks and do not complain about those three things.

4. Causes of Disease In Parts of Bone

Many people in this world have an accident then fracture. The man suffered from fractures is not caused by an accident, but the cause is the cracked or strained relationship with his brothers. Many people in this world get an accident but no broken bones. But if you strain your relationship, so you are vulnerable to get fractures, bone cancer or bone loss. Excessive hatred toward your siblings must be controlled, understandable, and forgive as well as join them with humility regardless of of your brothers attitude to you.

5. Causes of cysts and myoma

For those who are affected by cyst and myoma then keep a good relationship with your mother sincerely. Anyone who does good and attention for both parents, then later the parents in their old days will be really cared and treated well by their children and protected from the diseases in head, cyst and myoma.

6. Causes of Impotence

The cause of impotence disease is a habit when there are guests then they are not considered to be important and reluctant to meet. Our advice, if there is a any guest and any interest, gladly go seeing them. If you are in a state of fatigue then there is any guest, so compel yourself to see him happily, you certainly will not be affected by the disease of impotence.

7. Causes of Diseases In Part of Head

Whoever you are, whatever race, whatever the religion even if you are brave or prejudiced towards your father or your employer then you are prone to diseases in part of head (brain cancer or sinusitis). So, be kind, respectful, and obedient to your father or employer then you will not be affected by brain cancer or other diseases in the head. When, we get any duty from our employer then conduct it without any hesitation even if it is less good. The one taking responsibility is your employer when it relates to government and Allah Knoweth either the appearing ones or hidden ones.

The cause of sinusitis is a prejudice to employer or leader when working. Respect your employer as it should be, regardless of your employer attitude. Respect to leader is a liability. Keep your heart from any prejudice against leader then you will not be affected by sinusitis. When someone hates his employer then there are two nerves in nose and under nasal cavity coincide because there is one stretching nerve. This happens over and over again so that there is fluid buildup in the nasal cavity, in longer time, it results in an infection inside the nose called as sinusitis. How to cope with sinusitis is by remembering the leader kindness so the stretching nerves will loosen and be back to normal, in addition just get any treatment.

8. The cause of Tongue Cancer

The cause of tongue cancer is like talking about other badness (like talking badness).

9. Causes of haemorrhoid

The cause of haemorrhoid disease is if having passionate ambition without being aware that the outcome is determined by *the Supreme Determinants*.

10. Causes of Lung Disease

If you have lots of money and then are borrowed by others but then they do not return the money for a long time, then your heart certainly feel pain. The cause of heart to feel pain, is not because of money or someone, but the money ownership. Indeed, the property and children are the entrusted mandate. At such times, there are some stretched nerves in the lungs resulting into wet lung disease. When it gets severe, the lungs become swollen and by severe pain on the problem earlier so that it becomes lung cancer. Brothers and sisters, in every heart movement such as anger and suspicion, there must be one stretched nerve. When there is love in the impulse then the nerves will move in a positive direction.

The cause of lung disease is feeling uncomfortable and always wanted to be angry because the amount of money, property, or inheritance which cannot be returned by the borrower. If you experience these events then it will be nice to connect this heart to the Giver. The trick is to realize that children and characteristic are only mandates or the trust from the Grantor. If Allah wills entrust these treasures, so there will certainly be any ways to return them. Had it not through the people who borrowed that it can be returned through other people. That kind of thinking can make comfortable heart and feeling and be protected from lung diseases.

11. Causes of Appendicitis and Stomach Diseases

The cause of appendicitis is an attitude to be too anxious and worried about jobs, position, and finance. Instead, try as much as possible while about the number of results and when the results come, these are absolutely given to *the Supreme Determinants*. Being worried about job or position signifies the fear of hunger and not fear of the Almighty. Such an attitude makes susceptible to appendicitis or ulcer disease.

Therefore, do not like to complain about the work because people who like to complain whatever the reason is the same as saying that Allah tests his servants beyond his limits.

Indeed, the test is always given as the ability but the material unwittingly is the human beings themselves choice.

Diseases in part of the stomach comes from yourself namely the fear of income. In addition, that the anxiety of earnings is not immediately corrected, it can lead to ulcer disease, colon cancer, and appendicitis. Therefore do not worry about earnings and the most important thing is to do everything possible. Regarding the results, just give it entirely to The Giver.

12. Causes of Disease in part of Kidney

The cause of kidney stones is to educate children by hard way. In educating children, just try as fair and wise as possible, in spite of their attitude, their mischievous, rich or poor. Educating children is an obligation but if you educate children by excessive anger then the renal nerves will be stretched. If it is done for a long time then you will be threatened by a kidney stone. But if it is added with despair, so the kidney failure will await you.

13. Cause of Less Good Hearing (deaf)

The causes of poor hearing (deaf) is not because of age but the cause is that when you were youth, you less appreciated what was being said by other person. My brothers, take any lessons from it.

14. Causes of Back Pain

First drink plenty of water and then do not complain about your wife / husband and your children. We take care of them because it is an obligation and not a burden. If this is done then you will avoid any back pain.

15. Causes of Diabetes

The cause of diabetes disease is less harmonious relationships with parents and the unfair attitude towards children. If it is not corrected immediately, the diabetic will wait and no one will be able to escape or hide from the disease. The Diabetes disease is not because the diet but the cause is the mindset. The mindset drives the body, while the brain gets instructions from the heart. In the heart, there are four elements of creature, namely devil, female genie, male genie, and angels. The four elements are present in every human body and the most dominant in the body depends on the worship.

The Worship because of the world, then the most dominant one is the devil. The worship because of fear of hell, then the most dominant one is the female genie. The worship because of haven / intercession / reward, then the most dominant one is the male genie coming from the sun and worship for Allah, the driving force is from Allah SWT angels. So, whatever has been said is not without knowledge. The above explanation is to pray for personally *inna shalati wa nusuki wa mahyaya mamati –* *indeed that my prays, my worship, my life and my death are all for you God.*

80% of diabetes disease can be cured if you can understand and believe in two things:

Never ever think that diabetes is a hereditary disease. It is true that diabetes is a hereditary disease but the one is decent is the characteristic and not the illness. By understanding this, it is already a war and debate in your heart. The war is a war against your own desires or can be called as an instinct war against conscience. There are four instincts, while there is only one conscience. The instincts consisting of four core comes from the ground, core of fire, core of water, and core of wind. While the conscience comes from *lahw Mahfudz*. Therefore we believe that all human beings are basically good but because of the conscience, then they has been colonized by one's own desires (lust anger) so that it will be a variety of prejudices and conflicts. Then, it arises threats with no basis and colonize each other and mutually defend each selfishness.

If a patient thinks that the diabetes absolutely cannot be cured than he is positively not the followers of the Prophet

Muhammad. Although he is Moslem, but it is only a religion while his attitudes, traits, and actions are not Islamic. The followers of Prophet Muhammad certainly agrees with the words of the prophet that 'every disease has a cure, except senile'. Hopefully, in this world, there is still a doctor who is a believer so as to have the courage to explain where the Truth and The Falsehood. Being fear of Allah and do not be afraid of anything. Believe that the sustenance is from Allah and not from a job.

Thus, two things must be understood, although it is just a bit but it is not easy to do. Only people who have faith can do it or change its rationale. If one can change the way of thinking as above then within you, it will come out the positive elements / healers from the hearts.

16. Causes of Eye Disease

The cause of nearsightedness (myopia) as an eye disease is less attention to the close relatives. Try to maintain good relations with the whole family without any exception and regardless of their attitude to you. The cause of nearsightedness as an eye disease is less attention to distant relatives. Any diseases we get without being recognized or known indeed are our choices.

There is a story that can be learned: One day there was a cleric came to my house. He asked me about the cause of wearing glasses because in the past, reading Holy Quran without glasses, but now wearing glasses. At that time, I immediately answered, then he explained that it was no use to drink any drugs to cure my myopia, he told me that directly the cleric went home, should I go to my your relative house whom I hated most. When we got there, no need to apologize and just relax but the important thing was the relationship and did it happily, then went to other relative houses until completed. Finally he understood it and left the home.

Two weeks later I got an invitation of recital in Pasuruan. After the recital, I was picked up by two clerics whom I met last week. I almost forgot to clerics because he is not wearing glasses. By the time he was asked why he could recover and I answer because you were too busy with your bad prejudices with elderly relatives so was not even care to other brothers. Allah SWT loves you so that the vision was normal again. He had approximately 4,000 students. If less concerned with its surroundings, this will make the eye impaired.

17. Causes of Mumps and Lymph Nodes

The cause of mumps and lymph nodes are the attitude to be calm or careless when there is a little problem with any family member. If this is done continuously then there are two possibilities, mumps and lymph. You can determine the level of its severity on how much your anger is.

Learn to against your heart flush because the good and bad of the body depend on the liver. Therefore, in the Al-Quran, it is forbidden to not greet to each other more than three days. Until the fourth day, it begins negative process affecting on nerves in one part of the body.

18. Causes of Hepatitis

The cause of hepatitis is to hate someone continuously for a long time. Viral hepatitis according to common view is a type of malignant disease. I will give you the necessary measures for patients with hepatitis, in addition to the treatments. Look for a quiet time while you are alone and then find in your heart any people who you hate most. When you meet the people who do not like, then invite to shake hands and forgive his mistakes if the person has any faults, just do this to all people you hate to clean your heart from any hatred and revenge.

If the above measures done, then the vicious virus will be reduced approximately of 50% from the initial one. You should also be treated and brought to the laboratory to ensure that you are free from the hepatitis virus now. If you are healthy then, make it as a lesson for the future, just being kind to anyone and watch your attitude with others. The attitude can impact on your body health.

19. Cause of Illness in part of Knees

The cause of illness in knees is worry about the lack of capital and a close relationship with relatives, especially siblings. There is a story that a mother came to my house by holding her legs precisely at the knees. The mother was already suffered from pain in knee for one week. I suggested the mother not to think too much about the matters of capital business which had been determined by God while we try as much as possible and human has no dealt with the result. After I explained about the cause to the mother then she immediately laughed. It turned out that the mother was laughing while walking normally and did not feel any pain in the knee.

Once finished laughing, I asked the cause she laughed. It turned out that the mother was in a fight with his son about of the capital business before coming to me. My advice was to have no feeling to be unable to accept on the matters of wealth and children at her heart. The wealth and children were the mandate / surrogate of the Supreme Love. Never complain about earning and remain to be grateful for the amount predetermined by the Most Giving. We must try to avoid eating other property, except with commerce. Undoubtedly, your body will always be healthy.

20. Causes of Illness In Parts of Hand

The cause of pain in the right hand bone is less familiar with his brothers. While the cause of pain in the left hand bone is less familiar with your wife's sisters.

21. Causes of Pinched Nerve

The cause of pinched nerve is there someone being disliked or hated. Prophet Muhammad healthiness physically and spiritually were because he had nobody to hate. Though, there were many people make him as their enemy, he was full of forgiving and excuses for others. Slowly you will feel the beauty of Islam, just be the real Islam.

22. Cause of Prostate and Hernia Diseases

The cause of prostate and hernias disease are often being angry at mother and the person has many desires but he does not return it to The Determinant. The way to handle it is by being good to mother and get treatment. It is very important to know so that it can be a lesson for the future. Always read the two-sentence of faith confession in heart and read it because of Allah, surely you are in a state of physical and spiritual Moslem. Do not just have Islam as a religion but there are even no slightest characteristics or signs of Islam.

The process of Diabetes and Cancer Diseases

Every human body has a balance namely the feelings of joy and sadness, love and hate, as well as in the human heart, there are is prejudice and positive thinking. When one getting senses of love or hate then there will be two strained nerves. The nerves can affect on lymph circulation and one of the fluids in the body.

For example: There is someone who is in a fight his spouse and it is for long term consecutively. In his heart, there will be two strained nerves. The strained nerves in longer time will cause much liquid in the heart. The function of the fluid in normal amounts is to fix the heart, but with a sense of hatred then it creates more fluids so as making more tensed nerves. Such a condition makes the body feel tired and in the long term, get heart cancer or breast cancer.

Before being aware of the disease causes, although the disease has been in surgery but if one does not improve his attitude then it is most likely that the cancer will be back and may be worse. It is such a natural occurrence namely when there is a full moon that there will be a sea tide. The sea water tends to flow towards the moon. The is similar to those seen in the body that when parts of body are injured then the fluid is going to come to repair the wound. The causes of heart cancer and breast cancer are almost the same namely the prejudice against partner.

Someone thinks that diabetes disease is a hereditary disease then automatically the person is not wise to his children. A person suffering from diabetes in pancreas, there are two stretched subtle nerves. The first nerve leads to his own affairs while the second nerve leads to the children's affairs. The stretched nerves from pancreas is also handled by the body fluids so that it affects on two things: the pancreas becomes swollen or dries (wet-diabetic and dry- diabetic) so that the insulin production which is normally obtained from the pancreas becomes neglected and causes the unfulfilled insulin in the body. The problem is actually very simple to overcome that is by juxtaposing the two stretched nerves as by improving the relationships with parents and relations with the children. If this is done then the two nerves is normal again and the insulin production by pancreas is normal. It is regretful when the pancreas continuously exposes to chemical because the insulin production is not good as a result of damaged part of pancreas.

Someone who is angry or hate against his father by any reason, there will be a strained nerve in the head. The level of strained nerves in the head can be measured by knowing how the hatred towards his father. That is called by planting the seeds of brain cancer. We should apply the law as children to parents because Allah blessing is on the blessing of both parents. When we are dealing with children then we are guided by the law as parents to child whereas the wealth and children are mandates and trust from the Most Merciful and Loving God. The whole incidents particularly the bad events, the cause is ourselves while the good incidents are from Allah wills. Do not ever admit to something good because it has the position of the Almighty, and can be at risk of disease stoke. In terms of goodness, we all do not have the resources and efforts except by His will.

This body is from father and mother. When both are combined into one, then the body becomes stronger and can last from several diseases. Prejudice to parents can cause the body to be separated so that the bone is fragile, the flesh is perishable, easily get torn skin, easily get numb nerves, and possibly the part of body can be amputated. Most people with severe illness will think that it is a test from Allah SWT. It should be understood that all diseases come from ourselves and do not ever blame Allah SWT. As a Muslim, a person should be able to distinguish between salt and salty, between the sun and its rays, and between father and his characteristics. While one is emulated by people with diabetes, is not his father but himself. So, we should not be misunderstood as a Muslim should be able to distinguish between the Truth and falsehood. This issue should be clarified and reinforced by improving relationships with both parents. When it is done with sincerity, undoubtedly your illness will be cured before taking any medication.

The believers blessed by Allah, from the lengthy explanations which have been described, essentially our children later does not continue to have the opinion that diabetes is inherited from both parents. As a believer, we must be able to distinguish between salt and salty taste but the salty is not necessarily as salt. Similarly, the believer is definitely Islam but Islam is not necessarily a believer.

The amputation of chronic diabetic patients is from foot

The chronic diabetic amputation is started from foot because heaven is lying at mother's feet. Having any distance with both parents means to create a veil between children and parents. It will be a hindrance to heaven. The believers, Let us together struggle as our limited capabilities so that future generations can open their hearts. We do not feel tired of giving warnings and *mauidhotul tausiah* – good advices to children and grandchildren as well as relatives.

How to cure diabetes is that it should start from a belief that a disease is definitely curable and that the healing is clearly not possible chemistry but it is drugs derived from plants and seeds. The opinion that diabetes is hereditary and there is no cure, that this opinion is misleading. Brothers and sisters, that explanation is not something trivial. Do not see who is speaking, but listen carefully to what is being said and what is written about science. We do not have any resources and efforts for kindness except by the will of Allah, the Almighty. We all love the Prophet Muhammad then cherish and uphold high his saying.

We do not blame the people who worship as mundane, worship for fear of hell, and worship for heaven. Everything is true when children are not legally *baligh*-adult. While we have already been elderly and had gray hair but still like a child. We just know Allah only by His names but do not know Him. A person knowing Allah then he will not have the characteristics of jealousy and prejudice toward anyone and do not eat money recklessly except by commerce.

Causes of Diabetes is Not Descendant

One may believe that diabetes is a hereditary disease and diabetes insist that there is no drug for it. If thinking so then forever the person will never be a believer or his spiritual will also not be connect to Allah and the Prophet Muhammad as indirectly the person prejudices toward parents, and indirectly ignores or underestimates Prophet Muhammad that there is no cure except for the senile diseases. Al long as human has the opinion from generation to generation, though he kneels (prays) until his forehead is black then he still will not connect to Allah SWT. Diabetes disease is not a hereditary disease but the descendant one is the attitude or character and not the parents.

The opinion that the diabetes disease as hereditary making nursing homes more and more.

A believer must respect and uphold the words of Prophet Muhammad. We indeed may not hate the people who think that the diabetes disease is hereditary, but we are very sorry because one day in the last days, he will not be accepted by Allah SWT and will also not be possible to meet the Prophet Muhammad. The joy of the world is not worth of the pleasure to meet Allah SWT. Misery in the world is nothing compared to the agony in hell. Prophet Adam to Prophet Isa AS when collected together is not comparable to the Prophet Muhammad in every way. Therefore, do not underestimate his saying. In the hereafter if one is defended by Prophet Adam to Prophet Isa AS then, he still will not be free from the hereafter court, but if he is defended by the Prophet Muhammad then he will be freed from the torment of hell fire. Those who believe, all lives in this world just think carefully on this.

Whoever engages in speech or action resulting in the loosening relationship between children and parents on an ongoing basis, this will affect on a whole generation of mankind. It will be greatly terrible for people who understand the state of world. The damage goes far beyond narcotics, ISIS, or terrorists, but these do not mean that we agree with their actions. Do not make mischief on the earth. Earth is not damaged, but the occupants are indoctrinated which can result in the much distance between children and parents. My brothers and sisters, let us together think about this for the sake of humanity. My brothers, characteristics can be in such a way. A big influence to determine on whether quick damage or not on this earth is the intellectuals, scientists and noblemen. All these three are responsible for the safe and comfortable of this world or not. Everything must be started from ourselves.

Origins of Cancer

These cancer cells are derived from the earth core namely the core of land, the core of fire, the core of water, and the core of wind. All four are in every human body. In every human body, there are two elements, namely the good and the bad elements, precisely in every human heart. The process of releasing the bad is when the liver has no prejudice toward others then the bad one as gas goes out. The bad element goes out of the liver through the heart and passes the heartbeats and affects on the blood. At the time the bad element goes out then one's positive thinking will always be into negative direction. If the bad element often goes out in a given period of time in the body, there will be a little seed of disease in the body. The disease seeds will appear depending on who are prejudice. Without realizing the person himself chooses the disease seeds. What diseases and where it is located and how its severity.

In one country where there are few people who do not accept the government laws or regulations so, it will form a group opposing to the regulation and this will be multiply, even they plan to rebel. At that time, there is a mass or its own life and it will be getting bigger. The explanation is such a analogy of the cancer cells and the growth of cancer cells is identical to the example of the above story.

The way to overcome a cancer by medical ways means that there will be an armed and violent operation. Perhaps it can be an easy way for a while but children and grandchildren grow up someday they will likely make a larger group. The sense is that if the cancer gets in a surgery, within a certain period this will grow again and could be doubled.

The event above can be overcame by natural medicine. The trick is not by force but by approaching families and children with love and understanding and given attention to them. Slowly they will become aware and the country will be peaceful. The sense is that if cancer is treated with drugs so that it will improve naturally and do not grow anymore.

Origin of HIV AIDS Virus

This HIV/ AIDS virus is a creature not from the earth but comes from *Sufia* Nature which is precisely in the sun orbit. Such creature is an invisible creature which is visible. Such creature are in two types: the first type cannot be seen but can be proven and the second type is visible and can be felt. How to prove the first type is easy when you know the people are affected by this virus, so his natures will be strange. These natures are aloof and doing good in front of others, including his own parents but the person has bad intentions.

There is an example of the first type namely a good people according to his neighbors, his family and his parents. A polite person and teaching Holy Quran, but suddenly the person is looked for by the police because of the involvement in a bombing, then in his room, it is found the evidence of explosives. The neighbors are not convinced because the person is good but the reality is not. This invisible virus is looking for people who diligently worship but not because of Allah but his worship is for heaven. Thus, when the nature becomes hard, he feels as the most holy one, self-righteous, feels want to go in a battle-*jihad*, and feels that this will bring him to heaven. The second type is the HIV / AIDS virus detected during examination. The virus initially is spread from animal and the ones sought by this visible virus are that looks this is the nature of such animals.

My brothers the Muslims wherever you are, just worship because of Allah, and do not worship because of heaven. If worship is for Allah, you indeed will be put in His paradise as the origin of Adam and mother Eve created. If doing worship because of heaven, it means deceiving yourself and you will be disappointed at the end. Then, worship because of Allah especially for obligatory matters such as two-sentence of faith confession, prayer, alms, fasting, and pilgrimage when being able, undoubtedly the Sunnah worship will be sincere.

It is important to understand the holy book of Quran. Holy Quran is the holy book especially for those who are fear of Allah SWT in terms of the ban and conducting His orders.

Ebola virus and HIV Based On Belief Analysis

Ebola virus is indeed a virus in real verses of Allah SWT. Let us consider carefully the properties of the virus. Actually, the Ebola virus is not more virulent than HIV virus. The difference is that the HIV virus does not move in the same direction or move in any direction but the Ebola virus moves only in one direction, namely the direction of the blood and its ultimate goal is to move to the heart. Ebola virus in the blood leaves fungus in its path so that the blood vessels become thickened or freeze. When the Ebola virus reaches the heart, so the entire flow of bloods will be frozen and the heart becomes damaged. People who are affected by Ebola virus and died, on their nose, ears, etc. will leave the blood until there are no signs of life.

Ebola virus grows only in majority countries having a thought for coup. Ebola virus cannot grow in a safe and peaceful country. When a person's heart gets peace (quiet soul), it will not be exposed to the virus. Ebola virus is a virus living and being intelligent and having a high infectiousness but the outbreak is not merely spreading. The virus is able to detect people who have the same character with it. If there is someone who has the nature to oppose to his superiors or the government then he will be affected although he dresses like an astronaut. If he does not have the nature of opposition to his government or superiors, even with bare hands and do not wear masks then that person will not be infected with the Ebola virus.

So, this virus is the verse of Allah SWT as a warning to mankind that it has no sense of envy with the leaders. While the HIV virus will not be infected to someone who does not have the similar properties to the virus. Do not worry about the spread of these viruses because the virus spreading pattern is not random. If all human beings on this earth maintain a good relationship with their parents, the diabetic disease and other viruses will be removed from the earth by the Most Merciful and Loving God.

Allah has so much warning for humans, but they do not understand. Let us make the virus as a warning by not letting ourselves to have such natures as the virus because in the hereafter, the ones will be judged are our natures and not our realization / performance.

NOTE: For People with HIV / AIDS

The first step that you should do is not to keep any revenge or hatred for someone who infects you with HIV / AIDS virus even though you know it or not. The transmission process of HIV / AIDS is in the self-nature affecting on its virus coming into the body. Thus, the virus is called by a trait. The virus is not arbitrary coming from and will probably come without a call of nature. If the person who infects you does not exist then you will be infected from others. If you can accept this thought which has been described above then you will not be hurt or hated by someone. Also the ferocity of the virus in the body will be reduced by 40% and its development is also reduced by 40%.

The nature of a person affects the arrival of virus into the body without any notice. Once the virus enters the body then what happens is the virus detects a person's mind and even controls it. Therefore, just think positively then read two sentence of faith confession any time in the heart and reading it is not for healing but because of Allah SWT then the Supreme Healer will immediately help you. If there begins to be light in human heart then slowly it opens his horizons and awareness resulting the viruses in the body becoming weaker. For brothers from other religions, keep in mind with the Creator. There should be no hatred towards anyone and should not be any despair.

How ferocious the virus depends on how the ferocity of your heart. Therefore, do not blame the virus. The more you hate against the virus, the virus will become increasingly fierce. Meanwhile, you cannot hurt the virus but the virus can hurt you then think clearly. Based on our experience that the AIDS patients taking Kalimo Sodo drugs for three months, the virus is weakining and its level of ferocity is much reduced and the virus is not able to transfer to others. One patient who initially is with 49 CD4 cells / uL and then it is increased to 223 CD4 cells / uL within 6 months later then it is increased to 353 cells / uL in 5 months.

HIV/ AIDS Virus Resistant to Heat

HIV / AIDS virus resistant to heat because it comes from the sun. If HIV / AIDS is heated between one thousand until two thousand degrees Celsius, this will be considered warm by the virus. The resistance limit to the virus heat is four thousand degrees Celsius. The drugs that can eradicate the virus is a drug which can save the heat above the maximum virus resistance limit. That is why until now, no one can kill the virus.

There is one very unique herb because the plant is absorbing the solar thermal power based on the required dosage and immediately taking from the sun. If the plant is touched, it does not feel hot even when it feels warm but it is mixed with other ingredients and then consumed, the virus is like to be burnt by thousands degrees Celsius for four hours.

Influence of Personality Against Disease

Disease is a creature who can argue, has purpose, and can debate but all diseases are snegative. All types of diseases start from the magical land related to the concerns about possessions, a mysterious fire over concerns about a life partner, a mysterious water over concerns about health and unseen wind over concerns with the position. If we are able to control it then we become physically and mentally healthy. If we are spiritually healthy so we get physically healthy but if we are physically healthy, it is not necessarily that we are spiritually healthy. Therefore, there must be a balance between the physical and spiritual nourishment.

A person suffering from a disease, the heart and feelings are sometimes controlled disease. Therefore, when giving advice to any patient, it should be based clearly. In general, the patient is stubborn and selfish because of the disease effects. We cannot be angry at the patient as there is one thing controlling him. We are in quite a long time research on these things so that we know the types of medicines until all types of viruses, we know their nature. My brothers, always read the two-sentence of faith confession in heart due to Allah, Allah SWT will educate you on what you see and what you hear.

Allah SWT language is parable language whereas the angle language is the *suryani* language. The meaning of suryani is based on the language they speak. When meeting with the Arabs, so the dialogue is by Arabic language and when meeting with the British people, then the dialogue will be English. It is the same as the Prophet of Allaah *Khidr* who was using the language which is used by the one was in dialogue.

Allah The Invisible

Whoever wants to worship because of Allah SWT, it is undoubtedly that the person is guided by the invisible things. But if one likes to dhikr because of earning then in his eyes there is only dollar, dollar and dollar. By the increasing age, one is not even getting bigger fear of Allah SWT, but the increasingly fear of being poor and the growing love for world.

Allah The Almighty The Giver

Whoever wants to worship for Allah then that person will always be guided and will not possibly get any shortcoming and will always be grateful for His gifts. The conclusion is that if there are people who are always in dhikr for earnings, so it is the same as not believing that Allah is The Only Giver.

Allah is The Forgiver

Whoever wants to worship for Allah then that person will be forgiven for his sins even he did wrong things in the past and the present or later in the future. Ones can be done because of Allah are two sentences of faith confession, prayer, alms, fasting, and hajj when being able and do good to parents and parents -laws. These are called as main the obligatory, when the obligatory is done because of Allah so that others will be sincere. There is no other way or path other than the straight path.

Note that this knowledge is seen from the border namely the border between east and west, the border between tomorrow and yesterday, the border between last year and next year, and the border between the starting point and end point. Knowledge of the border is not limited viewpoint regarding the spiritual journey. When a person reaches the border, it will be impossible to do exceeding to the limit and can dialogue with various diseases and other supernatural creatures. Allah has set its blessings to Prophet Muhammad and his family and companions and their families. Therefore do not be hesitate to walk on the road that he brought.

The knowledge we write is the composition of the tree trunk of faith which its root is not on the earth but is in *lahw Mahfudz*. Allah is omniscient (for each person), any person who wants to worship only because of Allah, surely the person will always be told about which other creatures do not know. Notification is always beneficial for all mankind. Do not spend this valuable time to correct the other mistakes. Correct yourself to become self-conscious and finally know oneself.

Being Cured is Not For Drugs And Dead is Not Because of Pain

It means that when someone is sick then he is treated and healed, the heart must have faith that *he has healed because of Allah wills*. When the desired person is healed by the Most Healers then you will be met with the proper doctors and medicine. For more details, it is healed not because of any drugs and it is called a character toward Allah SWT. While the character toward neighbour is to say thank you verbally to doctors. Someone has a characteristic toward Allah automatically will have character toward neighbour. If, human has a characteristic toward others, it is not necessarily that he has a characteristic toward Allah SWT. Someone who is a believer then surely that the person is Moslem and if the person is Moslem, so it is not necessarily that he is a believer.

There was a person suffering from an illness then he was treated everywhere and eventually died. Then, his family must put their trust and should understand that Allah is the one absolutely determining one's age and we should all be sincere. It means that if at that time, he was not sick then he could also be dead in any seconds. If suffering from a disease then it is obligatory for the treatment effort.

Chapter 2: Knowledge in Having Certain Character

Way Against Arrogance

Beware of arrogance because this character may not come out without any reason namely feeling to have merit, feel to be better than others, feeling to be most handsome / beautiful, and feeling to be more intelligent than others. Among causes, the most dangerous one is feeling to have more knowledge, especially the knowledge about religion. If cannot erase this feeling mentioned above particularly feeling for highly knowledgeable about religion, it is very dangerous in the world and in the hereafter.

Examples of feeling to have services is that there is a worker reaching his success, later he bought luxury homes. Then, All of his brothers were given attention and given steady jobs. If you experienced something like this, so beware by the alternating of your heart. The trick is to return to God by telling yourself that all of the kindness acts which have been doing are because of Allah wills. If Allah is not desired then it will be impossible to do something good. The whole goodness are because of Allah wills and all badness are because of yourself. All certainly believe that Allah is Oft-forgiving, but forgiveness is not given before admitting mistakes. If recognition is often done so the characteristic of arrogant does not have a foothold to appear. Seeking knowledge is an obligation from the birth to the death, but the feeling to have more knowledge is not helpful.

Satan was cursed by God because of his arrogance by feeling that he was more holy than others, feeling greater, and feeling to be more knowledgeable than the Prophet Adam U.S. so he was cursed (the wrath of Allah). Thus, the most formidable opponent in ourselves is the characteristic of arrogant. Devote entirely to God then there will be the possibility to be free from the temptations of Satan and genies. That the application of paragraph *inalilahi wainalilahi rojiun*. To obtain useful knowledge then honor your teachers and do no prejudice them. In this world, there is no coincidence because obviously there must be any causes, but it is not easy to find the cause. You want your spouse to be nice to the parents in-law then be nice to your in-laws, regardless of their characteristics. Indeed, the day of vengeance will be started since in this world, only a few people who understand it.

Indeed, people are always complaining about the provision, the spouse and the children, unwittingly the person is cursing Allah SWT. Try not to complain with hard because of something happens now is for good. Remember and always read two sentences of faith confession because of Allah SWT. Keep away from arrogance and not to feel to be holier than others because the feeling will make your lips always cynical to others. The characteristic to feel the best will be fuel of arrogance.

How To Self Awareness

When we are looking at the wife, children, parents, or relatives who are angry, the heart do not connect with the last case because if it connects with the case then we will also get angry too. The way to overcome this is to connect ourselves with the Wise, the Most Compassionate. Tell yourself that one badness happens is merely because of ourselves while one good thing is because of Allah wills.

We must once see ourselves in a mirror. Seeing ourselves in a mirror then that we certainly see our shadows so we know something less good then we correct it. When this is concluded from the problems above, that we see children, wife, parents or relatives as our mirror and then what happening around us is just a mirror. If you want to correct, then connect your heart to God and slowly we can learn. Had our wives have always wondered about finance then the way to change it is that we do not always complain about finances. We must accept and be grateful for the salary / income earned. Undoubtedly, our wives will slowly change and they will accept and be grateful for the financial, exactly as we do. The cause that sometimes wife will be dishonest about finances is that the husband himself who is often dishonest about finances. It is impossible to not see ourselves stuck out our tongues in a mirror while actually we are sticking out our tongue. When we do not want to see the shadow in the mirror of sticking out our tongues, so do not do it. When we want our wives to be honest about finances then the husband should be honest about finances too.

When we are seeing our reflection by bulging eyes, then during the time, that the reflection will be in bulge eyes and no low will not be able to change it. The confession to God is enough by the heart only because it is your personal business with Allah SWT. When we are used to do it as described above, we can improve ourselves. We should not blame the people around us. We must try to eliminate bad prejudices from anyone so wherever we are, we can feel safely and comfortable. Personality can influence the atmosphere but the atmosphere can not affect on the characteristics.

Dear brothers and sisters, there are still many things we need to learn and we all should be able to learn self awareness. Whoever facilitate other people's affairs, the person affairs will be facilitated. Whoever likes to complicate the other affairs, it will not be long there will be people who complicates his affairs even for worse. When we have bad prejudice, then we will get bad prejudice too, and when we are in positive thinking, then we will get goodness.

If we are talking about morals then do not speak out other badness or can be called to correct others, better look at other goods or can be called as to judge others. Today, many people always correct others. At the end of the day, later the question is about our morals to others, and regardless of how other morals toward ourselves. Should we judge and not correct. At the moment we remind other goods, then undoubtedly the mood will always be good but if there is one in anger, then just remember Allah SWT, and say clearly in the hearts and lips, do not move that all goods are from Allah, while badness is this heart reflection there is still anger in ourselves.

In a state of upset or agitated, just keep silent for a moment and look in your own heart, who is the most people who you do not like / hate and just give any excuses for him and forgive him. The next day, go and talk to the people you hate most. You do not need to apologize but do good to the person. If necessary, just drink and eat the dishes served sincerely. That is how to apologize by behavior and not by words. After that, find someone else who you do not like, if he is not there then try to feel the burden on the heart, then it gradually will fade. Similarly, the condition of your health will get improved.

The moral applications above are not as easy as we read, but certainly we can do it as long as through the straight paths (the official *thoriqoh* or path by Allah SWT) brought by the Prophet Muhammad namely two sentences of faith confession, prayer, alms, fasting, and hajj when being able and do good for both parents and parents in-laws. If we have done the obligatory because of Allah SWT then the consequence is that the *Sunnah* certainly will be sincere. Had work will definitely be sincere with the results, if already married, then we can be sincere with our wives from all of his weaknesses and superiorities, and if we have children, then we will receive with full trust in whatever number and characteristics they are.

Obligations to Fellow

A husband must think about his obligations to his wife and children regardless of their attitude is good or not. When it is done, it will always remember that all wealthy and children are entrusted by Allah, and we can be wise to our children. We must think of our obligations to parents regardless of their attitude is wise or not to their children. Remember that the blessing of Allah depends on the blessing of both parents. We must pay attention to the attitude towards neighbors and relatives regardless of their attitude to us. That is called as self-correction and having no prejudice to anyone. Do not blame other person even if that person is wrong because it is his business with Allah SWT. We just remind each other with affection. My brothers, it is the intention of implementing the sentence tawhid '*lailahaillallah muhammadarrasulullah*'. My brothers and sisters, what we can do because of Allah are the Islamic laws namely two sentences of faith confession, prayer, alms, fasting, and hajj when being able- then, the *sunnahs* will be done in sincere. We must always think of obligation to God and to others, and do not think of our rights only. Allah SWT is loving and always keeps His word.

Angels later will question on our attitude and our responsibility toward our wife / husband, attitude and responsibility toward our children, and the attitude and responsibility toward both parents. Basically, one will be asked by the angel later is all about our attitude toward them, regardless of their attitude toward us. Whether they are good or bad and like or dislike us, but all is not questioned by the angels. Therefore it is not surprising that the Prophet Muhammad SAW said 'hold a law like holding embers'.

At this time, one place which is in rapid growing is a nursing home, so there also develops rapid diabetic. The cause of diabetes disease is the lack of attention to parents and children. Nursing homes are needed, but especially for ones with no family or relatives. Someone who wants their children to take care of himself, then no need to talk much to children. The trick is just giving attention the parents and parents in-laws even though the children do not know but Allah is omniscient. Later, the children attitude will be exactly the same to him when taking care of both parents and parents in-laws. This is called as the law which cannot be rectified. Never complain of any trials / tests. It is clear that something bad is caused by ourselves while the good is by the will of the Supreme Determinants.

By the time the bride will conduct the marriage ceremony, there will be a groom, bride, prince, witnesses and guardians. Then the marriage is led by the prince so that the wedding is valid. Whether the guardian in a marriage is clever or not, so, this is not the issue, because one is taken in a wedding ceremony is the person and not the intelligence or characteristics. It is a proof that diabetes disease is not a hereditary disease but one copied is its properties and not the person, therefore, do good to both parents.

If other people want to be respected then just respect others. But do not respect others by any intension, namely respect others so that they respect you. Respect others without expecting anything then Allah will pay attention to you and respond it.

Written Law and Unwritten Law

It is important to understand that the law in this world there are only two, namely the written law and unwritten law. If being caught in written law then it can be easily overcome with intelligence, eloquence, or are likely to escape punishment. But it does not apply for the unwritten law for the Day of Judgment which will surely come. No human being can escape from it. All humans cannot run and cannot hide from this unwritten law.

Sooner or later, it will come because in this unwritten law, the one who is the Judge is Allah and He cannot be influenced by anything and He will put anyone on trial as fairly as possible. Only Allah, the Most Justice One.

Our advice is that if you have no intention to be leader then learn about self-control carefully. The slightest goodness or badness, sooner or later must be shown. Keep in mind that in your chest there are your wife, children, and your parents as well as those whom you love, so be careful in carrying yourself. Your body is like a big boat sailing on the oceans and you are the captain. When you have been the leader, then the passengers are a number of people you lead. Therefore, be careful to bring yourself and always remember to Allah Almighty and the Greatest. We are really very small, let us together clean up this heart of hatred, envy, resentment, and purify our hearts from bad prejudices to others.

Proud of any mistakes is a source of arrogance, especially in making law, do not get out of the personal opinion but must involve many parties, especially the officials who have retired. This country has diverse ethnics, diverse tribal religions, and is not the private characteristic. This applies in making legislations such as education, health, etc. Therefore, an official should be able to release personal interests and prioritize the country interests.

One state is almost the same as one body. This healthy or sick body depends on whether or not the nerves are connected in the body. The connected nerves depends on its leadership. Incumbent President should meet more frequently and consult to the previous presidents. All decisions are taken on the basis of consensus and not of his own ego. In the new officials and former (retired) officials, it must be built good relationship - *silaturahmi* seriously if necessary, with the family. A great nation is a nation that respects its heroes. Leaders (the formers officials) are also heroes. Thus, the so-called heroes are not just someone who died on the battlefield, but someone who had been a leader (to fight for his country) is also a hero. When there are changes in the state regulations, these should be consulted to the former officials (officials who have retired) respectfully. A state official should know each other and keep strong sense of brotherhood to other officials as well as the officials who have retired. Let us build a culture of friendship, so there is no enmity between people. Realizing the national unity is the implementation of humanity.

When the above explanation is implemented, it will have a positive impact namely small communities are not volatile and the retired officials remain to have concerns for the nation. If the entire nerves are connected then the body will be in good shape and there will not be pinched nerves and no amputations. The meaning of amputation itself is fired. The meaning of a pinched nerve is that there must be no retired leader whose life in a bad condition. When it happens, the new leader must find out the situation and help them. The highest officials of the glorious country, when they meet the former top officials, then do not see at their ranks but take a look at their manhood and ages, you will undoubtedly grow humility. By the nature of nodding and saluting to their past as well as in the heart saying that they are also predecessors. Respect others with the same respect to yourself.

At the moment, we became leader when looking at subordinates then do not fully looked at their position, but look at their ages and experiences so that we do not overreact. If we become subordinate then do not look at the age and experiences but look at as a leader. Create an atmosphere as comfortable as possible in the work environment so that the work is not boring.

Procedures for Eating and Drinking

When we are eating, it must focus to the food eaten and do not forget to read *basmalah*. Chew the foods calmly and enjoy ones which have been given by God the Almighty. After food is chewed then swallowed delicately and stop eating before satiety. Then drink water calmly and say thank God, although by heart.

The meaning of the story is when we are listening to any lectures or *tausiah* then listen it carefully and do not comment. Then feel well and do not look at who is speaking but listen repeatedly to understand what is being said / written. When it is implemented, the food or spiritual nourishment will be perfect and beneficial for the health of physical body and spiritual body.

Mark of Prostration

Mark of prostration is a noble character. The implementation of this noble character is being devoted to parents, devoted to family, and devoted to the country but all of these can be done by being devoted to Allah and His Messenger. Let us all step on the law in a kind way to parents regardless of our parent attitudes toward us. Similarly, our attitude to others. The most important thing is that we have to be good to them regardless of their attitude toward us. That is called as mark of prostration. Thus, the mark of prostration is not the black forehead.

The mark of prostration cannot be burnt by hell fire. We have to be hard to our disbelieve characteristics and not being hard to other God creatures. If we are in a condition of many tests but we still have to worship to Allah then it is a great victory. Believe it or not that your will be later without any *qisab* - calculation.

Twin Suns

The events in this universe are actually a warning from the Lord of the Worlds. There is an event which is the emergence of twin sun. The meaning of this event is a warning to all mankind that do not discriminate between the stepfather and the biological father as they both have the same law.

When having prejudice to the biological father or stepfather then we will be in a danger of disease on the head. The force of law between the biological father and stepfather are the same. We should all be able to distinguish between salt and salty, between the sun and the light, the moon and its light, as well as between the parents and their characteristics.

Live and Life

Many people think that living in this world is together and when the dead will be alone. But for Allah is not the case, this life is alone and when the dead, it will be many brothers. The meaning is that when we will be the court of Hereafter, the complete questions are all about our attitudes toward our wives, our attitude toward children, our attitude toward parents and parents in-laws, and our attitudes toward religion and the country, regardless of their attitude parents us. Their good or bad attitudes toward us will be not questioned on the court of Hereafter. While, the complete question is all about our personal attitude toward them. Whether they are good or not, it is their business to Allah and it is not their business with us, the Allah justice cannot be doubted.

Note well the words of the Prophet Muhammad that people who are martyred, in fact, they are not died. Their spirits are in the stomach green birds perching on the lights and at any time, going up to the heaven. The definition of the prophet words is that someone who fights against his own desires (his own disbeliever characteristics) and not fight anyone else. 'Stomach of green bird' means as someone who is devoted to both parents, the belly is the mother while the bird is the father. 'Perching' means to be compliance to any laws at every step. 'Light' means to always get guidance. 'Any time flies' means to die at any time without any *hisab*- calculation.

Brothers and sisters, that is why, we feel scared when hearing any sound / events leading to the prejudice between children and both parents. Prejudice to parents is similar to close all the gates of heaven. Reflect carefully my brothers. In the holy Quran and the sayings of the prophet, 70% is parables. If you are much (little) understand the parables, you certainly will not be bored reading (studying) the holy Quran / Hadith of the Prophet. But it will not be possible, unless you want to worship for Allah. People who diligently worship because of others than Allah so, until the Day of Resurrection, he will not be able to understand the contents of Allah language (the holy Quran).

How to Take Lessons

People in the border areas of East Timor at long drought, it will be difficult to get water. They are looking for any water jerry can and taking as far as 3 km and they must stay in line for four hours. Water that they obtain contains of lime and must be strained before drinking. Nevertheless, they come home with water with happy faces and happy feelings. While others who are in the major cities with luxury cars and high incomes but they have face fierce and keep shouting to ask for a raise. Those of the opinion that the provision of a job is the real earning from Allah SWT. It will be nice to salary is discussed in a good way because it is an internal matter. The shame culture has vanished from this archipelago. Someone with many wealth, but often bribes officials. Supposed to be bribed and who accept bribes are equally given legal sanction.

On the other hand, we feel proud of the soldiers who serve in the border area. Indeed, we have great respect and high appreciation to the soldiers who eagerly help our brothers to find drinking water. It is a very noble act. At the time of drowning at sea, the used tire is more valuable than gold.

Greed cannot make happy but grateful for what it is and try to make happy.

Brothers and sisters, we must be good to take lessons in any event. Do not be bored to any discussion for lawmakers because the country is not private and adapts to Pancasila. When the laws are made by the interest of group, it will end up with riots. This awareness should start from ourselves. The truth is indeed embarrassing and painful but if want to receive it, in the long term the situation will improve. In the previous chapter, we explain the causes of diseases and many feel embarrassed. But the impact in the future can be able to prevent. Prevention is better than cure.

Wisdom can come anywhere, therefore we must be good to take a lesson. Lessons can be taken from any event or story. Most of you must have watched a movie called Narnia. In the previous chapter, we explained that there is no effect without a cause and no cause without effect, and there is not an accident without wisdom. In the Narnia film, it tells about four brothers in a conflict. When they are at a quarrel with their siblings, then the heart is controlled by a genie which is a characteristic of being arrogant. His men have human body but the head of buffalo and colonize other as well as are crazy for power. Old wardrobe in Narnia film is a parable of a person while the queen of genie and her men are the parable of our characteristics. Troops consist of animals and some troops are animal-headed man. It means that even though the subordinate is good but if the head is buffalo (animal) then all will be chaotic. Therefore, a leader must be careful and be wise.

When the four brothers had been able to come together then there will be goodness in their hearts so that there is resistance to not indulge in lust. The true troops are horse-headed man. It means for the diligent subordinates and wise leadership. The lesson is to establish closeness and familiarity with relatives and siblings, so there will be little possibility of any devil / genie to plunge us. Thus, Narnia film is huge lessons for people who know it.

Mahabharata is a long film involving a lot of players both in the Pandavas and the Kauravas. Pandavas and Kauravas are in the heart of every man. When the heart is lost by lust then the lust will be sat on the throne of heart as Dushasana but if we behave well with parents and respect to fellow brothers then the one sat on the throne is pandawa. Every day in the heart, there is Baratayuda war (war against one's own desires). Pandava will be powerful, without the help of their mother, Kunti and Krishna, so it will be impossible for them to achieve victory. Krishna is actually the Sri Vishnu who has repeatedly incarnated so they know about life and living. Krishna is the only man who has the Chakras and Flowers Heritage Wijaya Kusuma and insightful and has no other intensions.

All of the real story presently and in the past are the real verses of Allah. Only, humans can or not to read it. Remember that when the Prophet Muhammad in the cave of Hira and was hugged tightly by an angel with order to 'read !! read !! read !!'. it means that to read is not just writing but reading the atmosphere / condition and read the real verses. Therefore, Prophet Muhammad was instructed to read until cold.

The entry road of Devil and Genie Into Body
Ear

In human ear there is a road leading to a post. The post is located at the bottom of throat. The road is the devil or genie road when someone is heard unpleasant thing (news creating anger). By the time we get angry, the devil will open the door to get into the throat so that the throat will be tighten and make it hard to swallow. The devil creatures occupy the throat and affects on one's brain. The devil creature are in black false because the creatures are from the core of land and usually the person who are occupied by such creatures are the people who are angry about the wealthy.

If someone who are normally diligent to worship for his own personal fortune, so the door of his ears will often be widely open. If he worships for earning but for not personal (others), then the door of the ears will remain closed. The door of ear can affect on the heart rate and one's lungs. If the heart beats faster and faster, breathing becomes irregular and when talking, it gets stutter then upon such conditions, silence is better. By the time you read a two-sentence of faith confession in the heart because of Allah then gradually it returns to normal condition and the black creature has run out through the ear. If someone often opens the door of his ear then in old age, he will be affected by ear disorders / deafness.

Eyes

In human eye, there is a door and inside the eye, there is a road leading to Edema. Edema is located in the front of heart and in the edema, there is a post as a place for devils / genies coming in through the eyes. The door in the eye is very easy to be opened when the eyes are looking at something preferred. By the time the door of eye opens, then quickly the devils / genies enter into the Edema. When in the edema, there is devil / genie, the breath becomes unstable and the eyes will stare. In such condition, it is better to stay away and wait until stable. At the time the devils / genies are in edema, then there is only selfish characteristic and the body will be full of self-pride. When we encounter a person with this condition then, anything should be discussed because that person is definitely in the control of Satan.

If you always read a two-sentence of faith confession in heart due to Allah, then usually the person is afraid of you. But if you read a two-sentence of faith confession so that the person is afraid of you then that person will not be afraid of you. Maintain your heart and always read the two-sentence of faith confession as the first pillar of Islam so that it will avoid for doing bad things from ear, eye mouth and nose. Indeed, all four are from the bad thing in the hearts. Someone who is diligent to worship because of the human eye, the road will become bigger and the person will be prone for eye disorders, shortness of breath, and are vulnerable to heart disease.

Mouth

The mouth also can be an entry road for devils / genies leading to spleen. Satan / genie entering through the mouth does not affect on the heart and lungs as well as the person does not look like to be controlled by lust. Shaitan is derived from the core of water with the characteristics of love to talk but talk about the other badness. The person who are entered by such creatures will be happy to dig up other badness though in front of many people, it means the person likes to find and talk about the other badness in public. People like this are usually when he will be in old age, his name will not be remembered in good manners until the end of the world. People usually prefer to sacrifice others for the sake of lifting his own name. So, the evil devil from the core of water is even able to speak well and fine but there are intentions for his own sake.

In this country, there are many great people but constantly show other badness so that there will be no fragrant, meaning that there are a lot of great people but they always find out other mistakes until there will be no kindness. Satan from the core of water is white, so many people are fooled by his own eyes and not be fooled by their promptings.

Nose

The nose also becomes the entrance for devils from the core of wind and yellow. This type of yellow devils come into the nose and directly go to the heart. Someone will be easily accessible when he is diligent to worship because of long age or for position. People like this usually are proud of the people position and that person is confused and even prone to shortness breath.

How to Get the Blessed Earning (*Rezeki*)

Someone has a 1 hectares of rice fields and worked as usual. At harvest time, the crop yields for 10 tons of crops for many years and the harvest is similar to the fields next to it. When the rice field is sold to other person and the result is increased to be 20 tonnes by the same person who worked for the fields as the previous owners.

By similar way of working and in similar land but the result is different. This happens because the first land owner, at the very beginning, he had calculated the result and the harvest would be as estimated. This made little outcome and not blessed (quickly exhausted). While the second owner planted as usual and the matter of result was given to The Giver. This made more results and blessed one. This event commonly happens anywhere but, it is still not used as a lesson. The event is a proof that the earning is not from the field but from Allah SWT.

Correcting characteristic starts from oneself, family, and workplace. But no one is able to change it except for Allah. For those who want to worship for Allah then Allah will change it. If not worship for Allah then, it will be controlled by desires forever. *Besides Allah is anything but Allah covers on everything.* Everything is good by Allah wills and everything is by human badness.

Application of Affection

1. If you love with your heart so love your wife regardless of your wife love you or not. If it is done, then your heart will not be possible problematic. If you are less certain, then

careful for every disease in the heart, the person must have a problem with his wife or her husband.

2. If you love with your lungs, so do not complain about income/ earnings. Whatever the income you receive, you must be grateful. Suppose your money is brought by others, just give it up then let it go because then Allah will accelerate to get it back.

3. If you love with your own head, so consider and respect your father, even though he is probably senile.

4. If you do not want to get cyst or myoma (womb diseases) and prostate (disease of urinary tract), so do not make your mother offended / angry.

5. If you do not want to get into trouble on the part of bone (fractures, brittle bones, etc.), so strengthen relationships with relatives, either your own or your spouse. Regardless of their attitude to you, surely your bones will be strong until your old age

6. If you do not want to get any trouble on the part of intestine (appendix), so do not worry about earning, and the most important is to give the best effort.

7. If you love with your heart, so do no hate and envy to others.

8. If you love with your kidneys, so do not justify any means to achieve profitability. Keep well about what we eat and eat for your family.

9. If you love with your eyes , so pay attention to your relatives and your wife's relatives, either near or far.

10. If you do not want to be affected by stroke (half of body is not functioned), so get a close relationship with your own relatives and your wife relatives with all heart.

Chapter 3: Causes and Results

Causes of Rejected Prayers

The cause of rejected prayer is if you see a neighbour or friend who gets pleasure, you feel not like it, but Allah is omniscient either it is said or not. When you see a person in your level gets any success, let you also grateful for it sincerely. Then you will be more successful than the person in similar level. The acceptable prayer is to assume good faith to Allah and assume good faith on His servants.

Whoever likes to talk other badness, sooner or later he will get embarrassed. Anyone who prefers to give, he will be more likely to accept and always be healthy. Whoever plants the seed in tears and ran, one day he will harvest. So, this bad is caused by ourselves while the good event is because eof Allah wills. Therefore, do not commend yourself. Whoever please to commend ourselves in the near future, he will be drowned. And anyone happily praises someone, sooner or later he will be disappointed, then just praise of Allah SWT. Praising yourself is the seed of arrogance, praising other is the seed of disappointment, and the rightfully is praising to Allah SWT.

Our message is do not always complain under any circumstances because badness you feel actually is for your own sake. Try to be familiar with the whole family and consider them all. Do not always ask for attention or expect to get attention because it will make the heart miserable. If you respect others, surely even if you are old you will remain be respected by children and your grandchildren and neighbours. Just pray for your children and grandchildren as well as your friends. If you carry it in your heart, there will be a bit of peace. It is necessary to understand such characteristics, it is not performance affecting on the characteristics. If a person is good then that person tends to stay young and stay pretty / handsome. If at heart there are people who is being hated, then it will appear on the face and is likely to be exposed to severe disease. Keep your heart from hatred to anyone.

Someone who is getting trials of life but still read the two-sentence of faith confession in the heart due to Allah, and pray for Allah, even though he just gets limited earnings but still give the alms because of Allah, fasting for Allah though everyone does it for reward, and go hajj when being capable as well as being respectful to parents and parents in-laws then that person gets a great victory. A great victory is the winning against devils and genies. When being successful in fasting for the whole month because of reward, so the winner is the genie, but if not fasting then the winner is also the devil. Conducting the worship as Islamic law as a whole and because of Allah SWT. Once you died then in a state of prayer, fasting, and performing ablution and wherever you died, you will be included as death in the holy land of Mecca. Shari'a is the name of doing, while *thoriqoh* is the name of being done. If you go through the whole Islamic law as we already explained, surely you later are greeted the angels and none of the angels will calculate you because you are absolutely in the power of God.

Parent Feelings

Parents are people who have great services for their children. Giving birth, taking care, keeping, and educating with a full sense of responsibility are the parent services. By the time your children grow up, they are busy with their own affairs, so the parents will feel lonely. The issue we tell actually has a very simple solution. The discomfort is not caused by your children attitude but the inconvenience feeling is the expectation to get attention from the children. This is exactly what makes our hearts miserable and uncomfortable. Therefore do not wish to get any attention, it will be better if we give them the attention.

By the time, the sky is clear and clean of clouds then it will feel comfortable and very beautiful to look at. Every human heart has a heaven, when the heart sky is covered by clouds, it means that it is a sad time. The way to overcome this is by way of confession to God. How the confession is to say in my heart that the bad child attitude is my heart reflection, while the good child attitude is good obviously from Allah SWT. The genuine confession will make the cloud slowly gone, surely it grows bright and gets happy hearts. The sky is actually very visible on one's face. Do not ever acknowledge a kindness, because the kindness is on His will.

For those having many children, indirectly there will be a question in the heart whether tomorrow the children will be attentive to their parents. Unwittingly, a question like this is definitely in our hearts and it can create burden. The answer is very simple: depending on how your attitude toward your parents. Your attention to your parents will exactly the same to your children attention to you one day later. Do good to both parents regardless of your parents do good or not. But hold on the law of child to parents.

In Every Man Body, There's Universe

Out of many prophets who have only four companions is the Prophet Muhammad because in every human being there is universe. If we are being controlled by one's desire then there will be *Tha'labah, Qarun,* even *Pharaoh* but in the form of characteristics. Therefore, beware of the altering heart and do not be fooled behind any intention. The believers blessed by Allah, to prove that we all love the Prophet and love his teachings, we must enforce Sharia Law as a whole and does not undergo any artificial Thoriq- *paths.* Lately, Muslim condition is really in concerned because each feels to be the right one. If we are going back to the days of the Prophet

Muhammad that he was the only prophet having no students, meaning that Islam is a brotherhood.

Prophet Muhammad never fights against anyone, but he was being fought. My brothers and sisters wherever you are, if you indeed love the Prophet Muhammad then try to appreciate the friendship and brotherhood. We control ourselves and we think deeply on the prophet words carefully. Let us together keep the name of Prophet Muhammad to end all of hostilities. Live in peace with each other. Our true enemy is the devil and genie, and both are in the hearts of each of us. Therefore we all seek help in Allah SWT by passing along the way, and we all must be protected. Allah paths are two sentence of faith confession, prayer, alms, fasting, and hajj when being able. That is the meaning of the straight path going through because of Allah SWT.

It is truly devastating impact on making our own path (*Thoriq*). Yet, it is clear that Islam will not be destroyed, unless by the Muslims themselves. Nothing can be played off unless indeed the sheep. Whatever the reason, we cannot blame others and let us together make self correction. Clean up the heart from bad prejudices so, the good prejudice will be created and Allah will make it true. In the body, there are billions of cells whereas we have only one cell in the body of Islam. If every cell has conflict so the body becomes unhealthy. While the Prophet and his fourth companions are the heart of Islam. When

Muslims do not listen to the their voice of conscience then how will be Islam in the future. Let us together get self awareness (introspection). The size of one's soul is as big as RT (Neighborhood), as big as a city, there are as big as a country and as big as the universe. So he has broad horizons, nevertheless we must understand and always full of a sense of introspection.

One of human body is exactly the same as a solid construction and a four-story building. If the foundation is strong then the building is strong. But without a strong foundation then at any time the building can be destroyed. The purpose of the foundation is the whole Islamic law and executed because of Allah SWT. At the lowest level is inhabited by devils who are in the seven layers of the earth and its king is Dajjal. On the second level is inhabited by female genies who are in the middle of the month and his queen is Balqis Genie. There is one astronaut hearing the call to prayer on the moon. Indeed, the call to prayer is from humans on earth, namely the call to prayer from someone who worship because of fear from Hell and his voice penetrates up to the month. At the third level, it is inhabited by the male king genie in the midst of the sun namely the Ifrit. Whenever there is a man reciting the call to prayer on earth but the worship is because of heaven, it will be sounded in the sun.

On the fourth level, it is inhabited by angels and in the most central seat is the seat of the Prophet Muhammad along with his companions, Abu Bakr as-Siddiq, Umar bin Khattab, Uthman ibn Affan, and Ali bin Abi Talib. So, all men, there must be an element of devils, genie, and angels. We will determine in which level is our spirit. Therefore, if we want to fight against one's own desires then , we have to obey at one level until the three. When there is no single-or two-story building then people will not want to eat, drink, marry, breath, or work. If no two or three-story building, there will be no man want to go bed and awake. That is what we mean that in man there is a whole universe. Satan and genies are within ourselves, while we are not in devils and genie. When people lose with devils or genie, then it is not due to the clever devils and genie but because of the stupid human. That is why he is called a perfect creature, but no one is perfect except for Allah and His Messenger.

Cause of Family with Many problems

For those of new bride or groom, if once got closed to a rich, handsome / beautiful, and patient one but he or she is not your soul mate. Then remain to think that your soul mate is the one who just marries and not someone who you know first. In any case and whatever the attitude, apparently accept gracefully. In fact, there has been already a marriage contract.

That is the soul mate as the Award from the Almighty. Slowly but surely you will live happily.

If the heart regrets about the soul mate then it is the time when the devils and jinn enter your heart. Undoubtedly, you will continue to get whisper as always being problem. So beware of the voices in your heart (for men or women).

Causes of Chaos In Case of World Population

The cause of world population currently in a state of chaos is that too many people worship for other than Allah, one example is dhikr for earning. Actually, the person is similarly to one who do not believe that Allah the Almighty and the Giver and the person is the same as worshiping for the world by way of Islam. But they do not realize unless praying for other than personal purposes. Therefore, whoever complicates others, then his or her family will be as soon as get into trouble. Whoever is happy to provide convenience to others, surely these people often get unexpected earning. People praying does not depend on the verse, but it depends on the intention. We must be able to distinguish between Islamic law and Islamic Shari'a knowledge. People praying for others will get broad heart and broad minded. While praying for his own sake is enough in Fard (Compulsory) according to Allah paths – Thoriqoh - brought by Prophet Muhammad. Word of Allah *they seem to worship me, in fact they worship other than I, but they did not know'*. There is someone dhikr reading verses namely a letter of Joseph, but he reads it for women. By the increasing age, the person will not get the increasing *taqwa* – faith, but increasingly in love with a woman and also increasingly afraid to lose it. This is what we mean by worshiping to women using Islamic way.

The whole world already knows every concerned events in the State of Palestine because of the border. The incident is actually a warning from Allah SWT, especially for those who are Muslims as a growing number of Muslims whose deed exceeding the limits without knowledge. The incident at Al-Haram Mosque was the fallen cranes. The incident was not by chance but the incident was a stern warning to the Muslims that we should all be ashamed to God for worshipping is used as a business event. Hajj is Allah obligatory only once in a lifetime. Once go Hajj may be probably because of Allah, but the latter hajj may be because of who or for what.

When the sunset prayer, what required is only at the evening and after that the obligatory to pray is gone. Because the body is fit, then want to pray again and pray again, unless for *qodho* prayer, it is okay. But if there is no Hajj *qodho*, though at home, there are a lot of brothers and sisters who need help and many neighbors who also need help. Actually they are not deaf but cannot hear, they are not blind but cannot see. This is the impact of those who just think for himself. It does not seem to be strange for us that in Makkah Al Mukarramah, there was the event. We think that it should be a screening in each country to give priority to people who have never been to Mecca. When it makes difficult for people to pilgrimage for the first time, indeed it is a sin. But when prohibiting people who have been especially frequently pilgrimage, it is not a sin. My brothers the Muslims, discuss well and interrelated. Nothing cannot be resolved by agreement along mutual respect and mutual honor.

The city of Mecca is called as Holy Land, that is when we were in Mecca or at the Prophet's Mosque in Madinah when praying, give it for personal interests so definitely because of Allah, except for other than personal prayers. An example is someone who prays for his wife, his children, and both parents and to pray for all the Muslims and muslimah sincerely. That is called as the practice of *Sholihah*. But when praying for the personal interests and reading verses of the holy Quran until completed just for earning / women, so it is named as worship because of the world, using the Islamic way. The person in the hereafter will be placed in a much worse place than in a place of the criminals. Prophet Muhammad prayed until his leg swollen but he prayed for all people. My brothers , that is why it is called as holy land. There is not a place full of people with full of intention attached, if having any intention, better go to Kawi Mount.

Date Palm

We all know the palm trees. There were many stories that our Prophet Muhammad was under a palm tree. A palm tree looks very beautiful, its fruit has many benefits, and palm trees is resistant to weather. A palm tree has stems, stem, leaves, flowers, and fruit. All substances from the palm tree must have previously passed the trunk. All contained in the fruit must have passed through the stem. All substances in its leaves must have passed thought its stems. Similarly, the content of the midrib definitely must have passed through the stem. While the stem gets the content from the roots and the roots get its content little by little from the invisible land. Similarly, it is the religious life.

One lesson we can take is the Islamic law (two sentence of faith confession, prayer, alms, fasting in the holy month of Ramadan, and pilgrimage when being able) and devote to both parents as well as the parents -in-law (Trunk). All the five are compositions which cannot be added and cannot be reduced event cannot be changed. If there is one less than a fifth (Islamic law) if it is portrayed as a drug, then the drug is not a compound. All human beings are like leaves but as dried leaves because they have no trunk (Islamic law). Look deeply into the human body having a leaf (earlobe), fruit (breasts /

testicles), flowers (sense of gratitude for any gift), and seeds (eyeball).

On one trip, the Prophet Muhammad along with his companions met with one's grave who had recently died. Suddenly the Messenger stopped and invited his friends to pray by the letter of Al-Fatihah once then Rasulullah SAW took a leaf frond of dates to be placed on graves by saying, 'as long as the leaf is not dried then the death man will not get any grave Penalty'. After that, the group continued the journey. The meaning of history is that someone doing Islamic law in a whole because of Allah then the person will never wilted or dried. So, for more details, the two sentence of faith confession, prayer, alms, fasting in the holy month of Ramadan, and pilgrimage when being able as well as devoted to both parents and both parents-in-laws are the trunk, without this trunk then all the good deeds will be in vain. While the flowers and fruit will be obtained at the heaven.

Cause of Moslem Oblige to Know 25 Prophets

The cause of Islam requires to know the 25 prophets because in every human body, there is something from the 25 prophets. In every human being, there is something from the Prophet Adam in the form of the body. In every human being, there is something from the Prophet Isa AS in the form of the spirit of 'la ilaha illa Allah isa Ruhollah'. At the top of kalamullah, there is a nature called as the spirit nature but in the absence of Muhammad Light, then Allah would not have created the whole universe and its contents. Another name of Muhammad Light is the divine light. The difference is that the other prophets sent by Allah was only for one clan and if there are other people who do not participate, then they should not be considered as the wrong ones. The Prophet Isa AS teachings and his word sayings are correct. So, if there are people who blame the Prophet Isa AS teachings, it is the same as blaming the Prophet Muhammad as the Prophet Muhammad is not the prophet for the Arabs, but the Prophet Muhammad is the messenger of Allah for all mankind. While there are only four holy books from Iahw Mahfudz, namely the Torah, the Book of Psalms, the Bible and Holy Quran. The contents in the holy Torah, the Psalms, and Bible are all contained in the holy Quran. Therefore, it is called as the consummation. The fourth books are the word of Allah by the parables. The difference in Prophet Muhammad people and Prophet Isa AS people is so thin that when the Prophet Muhammad people with a mild tongue call the Prophet Isa AS respectfully. While the Prophet Isa AS people if they mention the Prophet Muhammad then just stop at the throat.

The real war is a war against self lust or desire. If there is a friend from one entity, village, or a friend from one dormitory, if he is in a fast increasing of level, then we must try to be happy and try sincerely. If it is applied in earnest then, it is most likely that someday you will be in higher level than the person. One prayer will quickly come true, if in his heart, there is a sense of pleasure when seeing other people get enjoyment. But, if there is no any happiness seeing other people enjoyment, then you will have difficulty in obtaining pleasure. Because one hinder your prayers is the displeasure and Allah SWT knows in detail the contents of your heart. That means as one's war toward his own desires. If you can win against the desire, then you undoubtedly will get higher level, have big heart, and be always stable when thinking. The real opponents for human beings are Satan and Genie.

Envy, jealousy, and revenge are the characteristics of Satan. While the feeling to be holier, feeling to be more correct, and feeling that someday will go to heaven are the is the characteristics affected by Genie. Therefore people in great worship and dhikr for heaven then, their speech and actions affected by invisible beings from the sun. And his name is Ifrit as a genie, which had once blocked the Prophet Muhammad at the Ascension. If someone who is diligent to worship because of the spirit of Heaven then he will be hampered by Ifrit men.

This World is Round

By the time you fly straight to the east then you will be coming from the west certainly. If you fly to the west you will come from the east. Similarly, the day of reckoning has been started since we live in this world. The meaning is that one who likes to complicate the other affairs then sooner or later he or his loved will get in trouble with the more difficulty. It looks like we are cheating on others but actually we are persecuting ourselves. It looks like we ease others but actually we simplify ourselves and families. Therefore, think on any action to be taken. No matter how small human action is, there must be a calculation, then do not think for a moment pleasure.

The world is indeed great as viewed closely. When the world is seen from the top of the seventh heaven, the world is no more than a tiny dot surrounded by light. The smaller one's soul, then he will assume that the world affair is big. The greater one's soul then he will perceive the world affairs as the provisions of Allah SWT. If Allah wants to give something to someone, so that there is no one who can prevent it. So, do not think of doing any cheat to get more fortune. If we do not cheat, the amount of assets will remain the same based on the provisions of Allah SWT. Only the difference lies in the beneficial or not of our characteristic. Nobody can escape from the day of vengeance and just wait for its time. My brothers and sisters, when you are getting remember Allah, you will be more able to control your lust or desire.

Looking for money is heavy and hard but in fact, the much more difficult is to put it into practice. If doing something is because the willingness to be praised by others, so it is easy but in the hereafter, there will be kindness for this but merely sin (called as 'riya'). At this time, we are concerned because it has become a habit that giving something must be documented (photographed or recorded), if not, so the thing will be not given, Brothers and sisters, let us always be alert to our own hearts. Maintain such intention and do not do anything without any knowledge. Useful knowledge can enter into hearts when we are humble. At the time of being high-minded, though one is not blind but he cannot see and not deaf but he cannot hear. Remember well that the real opponents are the devil and demons. Such creatures are in each of our chest respectively. Let us all fight against own desires.

Causes of Infant Deaths In Womb

By the time the baby is three months old, the baby is visited by an angel. Then the baby is invited in a special dialogue about the world affairs namely its earning and its amount. If the baby has agreed, then he will raise his right hand and say, 'Pas'. After that, the baby is marked by lines on the palm of his right hand or can be called with a hand sign. At the time the baby is the age of seven months, the angel comes to the baby again and then invites him to an dialogue again about soul mate and deal with it in detail. When the baby has been approved then the baby said, 'I received' by raising his left hand. Then the angel gives hand signs on the palm of his left hand.

In less than ten days before the birth time, an angel comes again. The angel invites him to an dialogue and discusses about death. Between Angels and the will-be newborn baby, there is a lengthy bargaining about age. It is the key moment because during day and night, the angel and baby are still in discussion and no coercion. If the baby has agreed then he will raise his hands, saying that, '*I agree*' and the baby is born on this earth. The baby is born with his palms open while crying. The baby's first cry is for forgetting about what has been discussed with the angels during in the mother's womb. While the latter cry is from the cold. That is why, regardless of the number of one's income then it seems always not enough. And how much income, it feels like being chased by the desire to feel not enough. Try to listen very carefully when there is a bride who is in a marriage ceremony, the bride always says: '*I accept.*' The words are the same as the dialog when in the womb.

Origin of Pocong and Hanging Ghost

The real ghost has no shape and its origin is from Kumoro. Kumoro is one devil who never stays long enough in human body. So that when someone dies, the creature becomes haunted. It is not his spirit exploring because his spirit has been carried by the angel into *barzakh* to be asked his responsibility toward his life. The performance of ghost embodiment is adjusted by the angels. Anyone seeing the *pocong* ghost, it means the person seeing it is always in dhikr for long age. So the increasing the age, the person is not getting *taqwa* but more afraid of death. Indeed, the *pocong* ghost sighting is seen as a warning from Allah but it is covered by fear.

Someone seeing hanging ghost means that the person does not have any the standpoint and the person always depend on others. In short, we know in detail the cause. Allah SWT has been lowered thousands prophet, has been lowered four holy books, and always gives warning at any time but only the person who does not understand His instructions. The assumption that the Prophet's descendants will surely go to heaven is very dangerous if it is not to be understood. The meaning of the Prophet descendants is not a person but the characteristics and attitude as well as conducting the *thoriqoh* or path brought by Prophet Muhammad. In these days, many people are making their own *Thoriq* – paths so that Islam will be classified in classes. Only the Prophet Muhammad who has the right to make the *Thoriq* because the Prophet Muhammad is the messenger of Allah. When others although they are great people but they are not a Prophet, they are only Arabs. Although this is bitter but still we would like to because it makes Islam a narrow-minded. Again, we say, do not have any role model or pride other than the Prophet Muhammad. Whoever he is, whatever his race, but Allah does not send any other Prophet after the Prophet Muhammad. For us, if only about a virus and diabetes, these are small issues. But about the man made *thoriqoh*, it is a very big problem because it can speed up the moral degradation process in the earth.

Cause of Forest Fires

The faithful humans always dialogue with Allah at all times through its real verses. There is an example of a country which there is a burnt forest so as to make people's views to be limited. Many people suffer from breath shortness and sore eye as well as many various problems.

The significance of the story is that the forest is the base. The base means as the Islamic law, the Islamic law is not applied in a whole fifth, then, undoubtedly the words and actions as well as opinions always make other people suffer and easily get misunderstanding between people so there will be understanding. And it makes people become narrow-minded.

Therefore, the incident is a warning from God to all of us that each person is not allowed to blame each other. The fifth we mean are two sentence of faith confession, prayer, alms, fasting, and hajj when being able applied because of Allah SWT. The Holy Quran is not a basic but its guidance for the

Muttaqin (the faithful believers). It is not the guidance for people who are afraid of being fired or being poverty. Stop blaming and let us self-correct. Let us unite together to forgive each other and understand each other. It will undoubtedly make a beautiful country just like a string of exquisite jewellery. Let us together love and keep this country with a sense of sincerity, mutual respect, and mutual honour each other and do not be blind to skin color or religion. Everything can be achieved if starting from ourselves, family, workplace, and society.

If someone has the above thinking, surely that person when staying in any country will make a safe and comfortable atmosphere. Personality may affect on situation or atmosphere. The characteristics affects on the performance and the performance does not affect on the characteristics . The real opponent is not human but devils and jinn. But the devil and demons are at the heart of each person. Therefore seek the help of Allah from the temptation to pass the tests, namely the Islamic Shari'a. If one can fulfill his obligations to Allah SWT then he can meet the obligations to others. A great nation is a nation respecting the services of its heroes. Great souls are those who respect others and appreciate their works. A person's heart will be peaceful and happy when no one he hates and not expect something from someone and appreciate them then it will always connect with Allah SWT. Do not expect any praise from anyone, even the self praise. Praising yourself is the seed of arrogance. While arrogance is an open way for misery, only Allah has the right to be praised. For those who believe, they will be very embarrassed when praised for they are aware that the goods are from Allah wills and the bad is caused yourself.

The wise man, if he loses something, so in his heart, it is not focused on who is stealing but focuses on the reasons why it is stolen and find the cause. There is a possibility that the money used to buy the missing items is money that should not be owned. Similarly, the incidence of forest fire, it should not be busy by finding out who burns it, but it is better to find the cause that there can be someone who burns it. One loses his money or a car, for sure his heart will be hurt. Surely, the one creating being hurt is not money but a sense of belonging. Where previously he is aware that the wealth and children are the mandate then if it is lost, he is not too hurt / soon aware. When Allah is pleased to entrust it, then it will soon be found or returned to others. Indeed, in this world, there is something missing, but all events are moving places.

Cause of Disaster

Had we let you know that Allah is Oft-forgiving then you will believe. If you want to pray for Allah, Allah SWT will forgive you and you will be given His forgiveness. All kinds of disasters in this world comes from the four core elements namely the land, core of fire, core of water, and core of wind.

In an area, there are many leaders conduct violations regarding the misappropriation of money / characteristic which is not supposed to, then it can result in landslides which can cover the road and disturb many people.

In an area, there are many leaders conduct violations regarding the misappropriation of assets as well as women, then there will be catastrophic volcanic eruptions and forest fires.

In an area, there are many leaders gather and discuss not too important things, especially to discuss other badness, then in the area, it will frequently get floods.

In an area, there are many leaders conduct violations regarding the misappropriation of position, then it may result great in cyclones / hurricanes.

In an area where people want to listen to advice / spiritual preach, then this area will not be likely to get any long drought. The person characteristics affects on weather and lots of rain does not mean as a flood.

In an area that is often cloudy but there is no rain, it means that people are in grief and always complaining.

In an area with changing weather (hot in a moment, then raining in a moment accompanied by wind), it means that all citizens are easily influenced and easily changed.

Many laughs in a short time will get sadness and balanced with the level of excitement. Excessive sadness will be complaints and desperate. It will be nice to be not too excessive and always grateful for favors given by the Giver. All the disasters in this world are only from the four earlier elements. For people who understand that, in this world there is nothing strange because there are clearly any cause and effect.

The Principle of Creation of Dogs

For people who know / understand that in this world there is nothing strange at all. Whatever your opinion about the dog but the fact that dogs are a creature of Allah SWT. The dog is *haraam* – forbidden when it is eaten and touched unclean but the dog is the real Allah SWT verse. When you see a dog then behave in simple manners and not to hate, and most importantly not to touch it.

This is a warning from Allah SWT that human beings do not have bad prejudices against anything and anyone, let alone prejudice to the Almighty Allah SWT. If there is someone who hates the dog, then it is not felt that in his chest there is a dog because the person is prejudiced, it is called a dog. Cleanse your heart from hatred to anything and anyone. So, more details what earlier forbidden are the characteristics if used by humans. The Allah verse is a warning to all humanity and it is not a verse for dogs. While the dog itself still does as it is. It is not easy to clean the hearts from bad characteristics and must be willingness to fight against one's own desires.

Meaning of Solar Eclipse

The solar eclipse is a natural phenomenon, but the phenomenon can only occur by Allah wills. Solar eclipse is a warning from God to all mankind on this earth. Solar eclipse has a meaning that too many spiritual human bodies are a state of fear. The fear is unfortunate because it is not the fear of Allah SWT but is fear of something obviously other than Allah. Fear of something can be described as the following: fear of being poor, fear of death, fear of boss / leader, the supervisor / leader is fear of being shifted by other candidates, and many are afraid of being fired from work.

While the religious men are afraid of hell. We are also afraid of hell but rather the fear of Allah SWT. Someone says something of truth but he is fear of not salable. A person will not be wise when he is in a state of fear. The above explanation is the state of creature as said to be the most glory on this earth and it is unlikely that they are fear of Allah SWT, unless they are willing to do the straight paths namely the Islamic Shari'a. When you apply the Islamic law as a whole then you may be fear of Allah (taqwa). The faithful humans can be guided by the holy Quran. Someone who is afraid of other than Allah then it is impossible to understand the holy Quran.

Chapter 4 : Message for Others

Message For Our Students

To get useful knowledge, the way is very simple but not easy to apply. If you wish to obtain useful knowledge then honour your teacher and listen carefully to what he says / teaches. Apply well the law of students to teachers regardless of the teacher is good or not when teaching various knowledge particularly the theology.

An examples of useless knowledge is that someone who is smart, clever and successful, one day become an official. The person is very honest but ultimately he is trapped by a problem and ends up in jail. It is such impact of useless knowledge. The knowledge is like a mighty stallion and when riding it and can control it well, then it will reach the destination safely. But if it is controlled by the horse riding then you will fall in the street.

One who respects others then the person will one day become respectable. Those who do not appreciate other works then the person will be impossible to live happily. Whoever likes to give difficulty to others, so the person and his family will always get in trouble. Whoever likes to facilitate other business, surely the person often gets the unexpected earnings. One who plants the seed in tears and ran then one day he will harvest it.

Message to grandfather, grandmother, father, and mother

For grandfathers, grandmothers, fathers, and mothers who currently sick or have bone ache precisely at each joint. It is not difficult to find the way of treatment. The treatment is by visiting the house of own brothers and brothers of your wife or husband. Be kind to them, regardless of their attitude to you. Although you know that one of them does not like you. And if they do not like you, it is exactly like you do not like them.

You visit them and stay in touch in good manner. You do not need to talk about the disease, but talk just the way it is and how he is doing, then after that you may go home. If your brother is far away then call on the phone and ask about his condition and so on. Then find in your heart who else the person who hate most, then contact him to ask for news. At that moment you will be healthy again.

Message For Soldiers (Army)

To all the soldiers in the whole world that what you are living right now is actually not a job but a dedication. In any rank you are, we think that it is something very honourable and noble. Keep your respective country and never get bored. You are the selected sons and daughters, respectful greetings from us, especially for soldiers who carry out hard tasks, remain in spirit. It is the right choice for those who become soldiers.

Our message is that if you have a duty to fight then you have to set the intention in the heart carefully. The trick is that do not ever want to kill your opponent, but try as much as possible to knock out the opponent and not to kill him unless there is intention and do not worry. In fact, the term of stray bullet can cause death but in fact, it is already up to the line that has been determined by the Supreme Determinants. Undoubtedly not by a war, the angels continue to perform its duties properly in the event of death.

By the time you are in a battle, just remember that your opponents are also human beings like you. He has a house, is awaited by his wife and small children, and the family always pray for his safety and he can return to the former condition. If you have a noble soul then you will not torture your powerless opponents. If a soldier goes to a war and he is in a great willingness to shoot his opponent in the head, then most likely that the person is shot in the head. The brave soldiers, just think deeply on above message and give cheerful face with big smiles, surely the country will also be smiling. Please accept our greetings to the soldiers / warriors around the world and also our own troops in the country, namely the beloved Indonesia Raya beloved and peace for our country.

Good intentions and positive thinking if they are done so in the short term or in the long term, then it will surely grow kindness to the children and grandchildren. Indeed, in this world nothing is lost, but all that happened is moving place. Respect your elders, and honour the ones who are retired earlier. Let us restart a great nation which is a nation with respects to the hero services, both living and died before us. The problem about earning should not be referenced and believe that the earning comes from God the Almighty. Whatever the amount of income, just receive and enjoy gracefully. The human happiness does not come from more or less wealth. Many people are with abundant treasure but they are suffering and many people are with few possessions but they are still happy.

The soldiers who serve in the border area is quite hard. The task is a noble task. When they are on duty in the border are, they may sometimes feel bored. The way to overcome boredom is that you have to adapt to the local community, both in the country itself and in neighbouring countries. The task of soldiers is to protect the weak and defend that right based on the country law and religious law. The soldiers will not be afraid of miserable and will not take one-side and he is always happy when he sees others getting enjoyment.

Keeping the border must be with a sincere heart and not the intention for promotion and not ask for the attention from the center. The soldiers will guard the border with discipline and check on the border zone and give attention to his family. These such soldiers are obviously going cared for and protected by the Almighty. Therefore do not worry about any things, Allah will pay dearly for it and it is not just given to you yourself but to your descendants that they will receive His blessings. Probably not many people who know about it but do not let your heart to complain. You should be grateful because not many people get a chance like you. Do not imagine the luxurious life because someday you will get disappointment. When others has a chance for devotion to homeland. Do not forget to always worship for Moslems. Always pray for the family and parents as well as your commanders. Obey and being compliance to your commander orders, your services are known in detail by Allah SWT. Whoever is expecting praise, he will get disappointment. Whoever is on duty sincerely, he will receive the glory. The border guards are the honourable soldiers, in any event they have to be very clever to take any lesson. Wherever you are, always give positive thinking to others, so there will be no badness.

Message For Teens

Every teenager in his heart always certainly wants to know who his partner later and how will be the prospective partner later. The answer is simple that, he is exactly like you. That is, supposed you like being mischievous to others, then your spouse is also mischievous. When, you like playing with women then your partner also likes playing with men. Consider the fine words of Allah: nd as of His Signs, He created mates for you from your souls that you may find rest in them. And He put between you love and mercy (compassion). Most surely there are Signs (proofs) in this for a people who reflect (reckon). (Letter of Ar. Rum 30:21). The purpose of the description is the spiritual body and not the physical body. If it is physical so, it is certainly not the similar kind but, the opposite sex. Had male monkey would definitely get a female monkey. Suppose there is a beautiful but kind tiger, the male monkey certainly will not have the guts to approach him. So, nothing to worry about soul mate.

clearly it has the preparation and clearly by no defects. Our point is that if Allah really wants, then you is definitely pleased and will not be able to blame your spouse and all looks perfect under any circumstances. He will still look gorgeous even if you look at him at his waking time and remains beautiful even though you see him while sleeping and everything looks by no defects. So, keep good care of your contacts if you want to get a good soul mate. Instead of body movement, even the heart movement has a calculation.

Message For Criminals

To robbers, thieves, fraudsters, gangsters, gamblers and criminals that we respect. We think that you are not actually evil creatures. It is just that your condition is being controlled by your own desires. We believe on your own heart, also realize that the acts are not good deeds, it is the conscience. But the voices of conscience are covered by negative desires driven by the driving force of anger appetite.

The way to fight against the prohibited characteristics by the Almighty is clearly s to start reading two sentence of faith confession in your heart, even though there is any problem or no problem and read them because of Allah SWT. Then conduct prayer and try to complete for the five times. Slowly the characteristics of want to steal, pick pockets, and commit other crimes will be reduced. How your feel is if your mother is picked her wallet, then just do what we have informed and the most important is always reading two sentence of faith confession and do not leave it even for a while. Allah is Oft-forgiving, anyone who worships because of Allah SWT, then Allah will forgive him. Oppose your lust and stop doing badness. Let us together maintain convenience wherever we are and listen to carefully your conscience.

Message For Students and Workers

Our message for students who are learning on religion knowledge in any country. Our message is to respect the clerics or religious teachers and not to have prejudice on them. Learn diligently at young age so then the knowledge will be useful. Obey to what he said, but about worship, then just worship because of Allah SWT merely. The worship because of the prophets is a wrong worship because it is just because of Allah SWT. If it is for others (non-private) then it is all up to you. An example is when the exam, just being diligent about learning and worship, these are because of Allah SWT. But if there are relatives who will get any exam, then pray for them to pass the exam. That is called as good actions. always remember to God and do not forget to pray for both parents and clerics who you all gain the knowledge. Hopefully, you gain useful knowledge.

The way to obtain beneficial results and blessings for workers is do not think of your own purposes when working even though you are in need of money. Think about the employer / customer interests and then work with your obligations well. If you think of the employer / customer interests, undoubtedly your needs are guaranteed by the Most Giving One. But if you are selfish, the results are likely to get less blessings even it will be gone soon, as water is placed in a bamboo basket. Everyone must know soldiers. They become soldiers together, are with similar wage, and similar rank. But, in five years, so some of them will have house, have married, and some still have nothing event get many debts. The cause is that the soldier at the beginning has the intention to dedicate himself for his country with sincere results so that this will taste good. But, for them with the intention to get much money, so the result can be so disappointed until reaching the point of boredom.

Message for New Bride and Groom

Within every human chest, there are five rooms, the first room is slightly black color, and in the room there is a kind of office keeping data about the characteristic entrusted to you. In the room, there is a note of the characteristic origin and usefulness. Everything is recorded neatly and correctly.

The second room is in red. There keeps pictures and names of people you love and their stories. If you just has been in a marriage ceremony, in the room there is your invisible wife or husband. Give him a respected position in your heart and do not let anyone else get in. Although you once knew anyone else but that person is not your soul mate. You have married a mate who is given by God and he or she is your soul mate also by her or his performance and characteristics. Thus your partner will feel comfortable and happy. When a husband does it then the wife also follows it.

The third is a quasi-white colored room. In the room, there is a record of all knowledge but only the records on the knowledge you have accomplished because the room is not included in the agreement when you were in the womb. For more details you should seek knowledge. That is why seeking knowledge is an obligation to enter the pit.

The fourth room is the quasi-yellow colored room. In the room, there is a note on the positions. Therefore, do not envy about the position. Although in the childhood, one was a poor child and also not so clever. But in his chest, particularly in the fourth room colored in yellow, there is a record of being a president although others agree or not and like it or not, he will remain to be appointed as a president. So, if there are people who are envy or prejudice to him such as people have prejudice toward him that he goes to paranormal, he cheated, etc then those who argue do not have faith. When those who believe if one defeats in an election, in his heart then immediately having thinking that he actually loses since he gets lack support or there is one cheating but certainly, Allah does not want him to win the election. In addition, there is no record in me, this is all for my own good. So in the one's heart there is no anger or hatred. When seeing from ability, he is superior to his opponent. *Those who do not accept My provisions, whoever is ungrateful for My gifts, and anyone who cannot wait on My tests and then just go out from My earth, go out from My sky, and seek God besides Me (Hadith Qudsi).*

The fifth is the main room in the fourth floor named as 'Qalbu'. The leaders there have the same appearance as you when were between 21-27 years old. They are dressed all in white, always smile attentive, loving, never talk any useless things, never speak other badness, being fragrance, all beings honor him even the angels, very calm, there is no sense of jealousy, and no sense of fatigue and boredom. At the surrounding there are four loyal aides, they have the same attention. The four are respectful and *tawadhu* - humble. He is actually a creature with the highest degree in Allah SWT side. That is the light of Muhammad used to be a man and for 63 years living in the earth, namely the Prophet Muhammad.

He died at this time and became the *mutmainah* desire who can stay in the holy body and live in the believer hearts. The Prophet said: even if you are happy to me, but not happy to one of my friends then you are not my class. Therefore, not only proud of one class only. We must respect the same for *Abu Bakr as-Siddiq, Umar bin Khattab, Uthman ibn Affan, and Ali ibn Abi Talib* and the other companions. Do not be proud of the descendants because it can make to be unwise. If a son's thief wants to worship because of Allah, then He will receive the help in the hereafter.

By the time the spirit is still alive, the body is the spirit clothes. At the moment, the spirit is already out of the body (died) then the *mutmainah* desire is the spirit clothes. The *mutmainah* desire which we described earlier is your form when between 21-27 years old or the time, when you were the most handsome and beautiful. That is called an angel, so an angel is your own wife in holy conditions then it is the embodiment of heavenly beings.

The holy condition is a condition where in your heart always read two sentence of faith confession as the first pillar of Islam because of Allah and then legalized by praying for 5 in times a day, giving alms, fasting in the holy month of Ramadan, as well as hajj when being able because of Allah SWT. When the five things are done because of Allah then it will turn out to be holy condition. The whole angels there will all be less beautiful than your own wife. Because to be holy, it can only be passed with *thoriqoh* namely whole *Islamic law* and there is no other Thoriq, except the *thoriqoh* brought by the Prophet Muhammad.

Islam is prone to any fragmentation because people make their own Thoriq. The only authorized Prophet Muhammad could bring the Thoriq of Allah SWT. This information is very bitter but must be conveyed. It is better than later your spirit will be naked.

How Bathing Baby Correctly

Water has its own laws and do not care about the others, namely the water moves to a lower place. The wind also moves based on its law and does not care about the others and moving in all directions. Fire / heat has its own laws and disregard the others, it is moving upwards or heating what on it although there are securities, the fire will continue to burn. Land also has its own laws and do not care about the others, namely if it is organically fertilized so, the plants will grow fast and continuously to get chemical fertilizers when, there are more ferocious insects.

If already understand the description above, how to bathe the baby well is as the following:

1. Open the whole baby clothes and prepare the water in the tub.
2. Get wet at the baby's foot then continue to wet to the knees.
3. Get wet on the baby's knees to the upper part until evenly
4. Soap baby gently until evenly
5. Flush gently with soap foam is clean
6. Once the baby clean, put the baby into the tub, but not for too long
7. Lift the baby out of the tub to remove water by wearing a towel
8. Close the baby's body with a towel.

The wet feet by water makes the body move up and bring winds in the body as the heat continues to move upward until it somes out. After the bath, the body will feel fresh. The above story means as a notice to clerics / scholars who give *tausiah* (spiritual teaching). The trick must start from the bottom and slowly, lovingly. Undoubtedly it can make the congregation feel the spiritual teaching given. When clerics are giving tausiah, the feeling must be sensitive whether what is given is true from the Al-Quran, Hadith, or as impingement for the feelings (disappointment). When there are something dislike, usually it can be such impingement for the feelings (disappointment). Purify your hearts from hatred to anyone. Every moment, there is a war between the faith characteristics and disbeliever characteristics. The war is not a war against the disbelievers but against the disbeliever characteristics. That is called as *jihad*.

How To Overcome Fussy Toddler at Night

For young mothers who only has just had a baby. Sometimes our children in the middle of the night are fussy and always crying. In the event, do not panic and do not blame your husband / wife. The way to overcome this problem, namely:

1. First, you find the pan (a container for cooking) and then put oil in it and turn on the stove over low heat.
2. The second step, you cut the leaves of onion in two or three stalks with nails and do not cut with a knife.
3. The third step, put the onion leaves which have been cut into the pan until fragrant but not until charred and then turn off the stove and let the onions warm / cold.

4. The fourth step, gently wipe with a red onion with a hand on the child's back and gently flatten the entire back then gradually your child will fall asleep.

There is something necessary to be understood that if you have many children, the children certainly have the most mischievous and annoying. But it remains to be wise on your child and do not discriminate between your children. Because most likely one day later after your child is an adult and you are old, the most mischievous child will be the children who most concerned about you. There are many such stories, then be fair to your children.

Benefits and Uses of Papaya Trees

For those living in rural areas, particularly for the ones with poultry (chickens) hobby. When the seasons change usually there are many sick chickens or cached jammed. If you are a creative person then you can make the medicine. Having many poultry, you should learn well how to make the medicine. How to make medicine for poultry is as the following:

Tools and materials :
1. 1 kg of papaya leaves (do not use the dried leaves)
2. Bran about 3 kg
3. 5 litters of water
4. Wooden ladle
5. Containers

6. Stove
7. Pan

How to make:

1. Boil the leaves of papaya with 5 liters of water until the leaves are soften and water is just a half.
2. Put the boiled papaya leaves with the remaining water into the container.
3. Then stir with a wooden ladle until blended
4. Once the ingredients have been flat then let stand until warm
5. Give the ingredients if the chickens are sick
6. Give the medicine in the morning and evening for 3 consecutive days, the poultry will be healthy again.

If there is a jammed cached, then do not immediately give directly the medicine above, but take the processed papaya leaves and then give it to the poultry. Wait until the birds are hungry for feeding. The poultry (chicken) is healthy when fed as described above, it will not hurt at the changing seasons.

How to make medicine for livestock (cattle, goats, horses, chickens, etc.) is as the following:

Tools and materials :

1. 1 kg of papaya root
2. 10 kg of papaya trunk
3. 3-4 kg of papaya leaves

4. Pan
5. Oven
6. Knife
7. Scale
8. Tool pounder

Ways of making :
1. Take papaya roots and stems of about 30 cm
2. Peel the skin until it looks greenish color
3. Weigh for 10 kg
4. Grind the papaya trunk and papaya leaves by grinding them
5. Boil papaya stems and papaya leaves until smooth but not add with water
6. Once the ingredients have been a little dry out by boiling, then put the ingredients in an oven with a temperature of 60° C until dry.
7. As it dries, grind again until smooth
8. Herbal remedies for cattle are ready for use

For those having a lot of cattle, it will be good to plant papaya trees. Papaya tree can be used to make natural animal medicine. When you will make the natural animal medicine, in making it, do not put the ingredients (papaya trees) in an oven with temperatures above 70° C because it can reduce the active substances. The papaya trees, in the period leading to bear fruits, have the best active substances and ready to be used for the making natural medicine for cattle. All parts of papaya tree (roots, stems, and leaves) will not be wasted because all parts can be used for the making the natural medicine for cattle.

The natural medicine for cattle when it is consumed by chickens, goats, and cattle, then the animals will be healthy and have fragrant meat (especially goat because it has unpleasant smell) and the meat is not perishable. My brothers, do not overly rely on chemical drugs; you do not only have to buy the chemical one, but also by the natural medicine, it will make higher meat quality than using the chemical medicine. Healthy meat for human consumption will be healthy for the body. Think about this for longer time especially about the impact on mankind and the children as our descendants. For those who are used to consume chicken meat, it is better to firstly boil the chicken with coconut water because it can dissolve the negative contents, can at least reduce the amount of saturated fat. Once the chicken is boiled then you can cook it according to your taste. As already described above, it is one way to maintain the family health.

If making the natural medicine with papaya tree materials is processed in a modern way and without preservatives so, it can be for human consumption because it is beneficial to dissolve the preservatives in our body and can be consumed by children and adults. You already know that the food and drinks today can almost be said to be a lot more harmful than being good. We can only try to minimize it. My brothers really, death is not because of illness but maintaining health is such an obligation-*fardhu kifayah* for mankind.

Death Process

The death people, in less than a thousand days, in the body, there is an invisible thing coming out with color quasi-black. Then less than a hundred days, then it comes out again the quasi- red color invisible thing. Less than forty days, it comes out again the quasi-white color invisible thing. Less than seven days, it comes out again the quasi- red color invisible thing. On the day of death, it comes out of the person spirit. Upon the spirit release, we cannot reduce and cannot be add the time. The time for releasing the spirit has been determined by the Most Determinant One when we were in our mother's womb. Time is already defined but the way of death depends on each individual behavior.

If reaching the predetermined line since before birth regardless of agree or not, the death will still be done. In the womb, there was an agreement between the baby and the angel on three conditions, namely fortune, marriage, and death. If one of these three things did not reach an agreement or not approved then the baby will die in the womb. Both parent attitudes or behavior are very influential on the baby agreement. At the time of marriage, the two read two sentence of faith confession and it is the embryo of conscience (spiritual). While the embryo for the instinct (physical) is when the parents are having sexual intercourse. So, if a child is born into the world without any marriage ceremony (*akad nikah*) it is likely that the baby will have no conscience (will not be able to receive helpful advice) and will be very interested in the useless advice and its habit is criticizing others, has feeling to be the strongest, and feel superior.

If the father and mother are married (special for Muslims) when a child is born, so the baby has great chances to become *Fitrah* – Holy and certainly has a conscience. That is called as oneself, so it is very easy to correct yourself and easy to be aware of bad behavior and feeling bad. People will not recognize the good behavior because they know that the good behavior is by Allah will. If the father and mother do not do the marriage contract so when the child is born without sin, it has no conscience and only cared about the instinct. While the conscience just feel to be better than others. Instincts can be called by *me* and the children are always aware of goodness or realize the position of the Almighty. As well as any acts, when it is applicable (being recognize), then it will be worthless in Hereafter court.

My brothers, do not argue that the one which can cure is medicine, but healing is because of the Almighty. It means that if Allah wants to heal someone then, he will find the healing medicine. It is very important to understand so that we are not being arrogance. It is also important to know that all the attitude and behavior eventually getting the Wrath of Allah or who make mischief on earth begin from arrogant characteristic. It applies to all human beings without exception to any nation and any religion. If each person understands this, so this world will be safe and peach. There will be no revenge, no envy and no prejudice. The above explanation is the meaning of war against own desires.

Light of Muhammad

The light of Muhammad is descended to earth, namely the character of the Prophet Muhammad. When the Prophet was death, the light of Muhammad which has been taught in human form for 63 years was being a desire named as the *mutmainah* desire. When a mother and father are married and firstly have sexual intercourse yet, at that moment, Allah set up a desire, namely the *mutmainah* desire, but it is still in the Azali Nature. By the time the father and mother have sexual intercourse then in the womb there is a desire, that is the desire of anger (when it has been an embryo). In forty days, it has been a clot; in the following forty day, it has been a lump of meat.;, in the following forty days, the spirit gives a life so that there is life in the womb. At nine months and ten days, the baby is born in a state of purity or innocence. When the baby is given name, at that time the *mutmainah* desire is put into the baby. After the *mutmainah* desire unites with the baby, so it is called as *holy*. At the holy condition, believe it or not, when the baby is dies, then it will not bring into the calculation process (hisab).

After the child is *baliqh*- adult, he starts to misbehaving, starts to have a sense of envy, and starts to be vengeful then gradually the *mutmainah* desire of this heavenly being will not bear staying in the body, by these characteristics, so the *mutmainah* desire goes back again to the Azali Nature. At not holy condition, then the words and actions as well as opinions, there must be any intension. Although one is diligently pray because of something and basically, praying is for one benefit. Though Allah the Adjusting but why we set it up. The Prophet Muhammad SAW was a very diligent prayer, but he prayed for his people and not for himself. To be in holy condition again, there is no other way and no one else except by passing the *thoriqoh* (Islamic Law) in a whole, namely two sentence of faith confession, Prayers, Alms, Fasting in the holy month of Ramadan and the hajj when being able. If the five things are done because of Allah so, the Sunnah practices can be done sincerely just because of Allah, *lillahi ta'ala*. The *Islamic Shari'a* is the top cause, while sincerity is the peak effect.

Someone who is every day in dhikr due to his own personal fortune by the increasing age, the person will not get the increasing *taqwa* - faith. The person gets older by having the characteristics of more loving to the world and getting afraid of being poor, and certainly being worse then, ultimately afraid of being poor as well. Someone who diligently prays for a long life but then he cannot increase his *faith* - taqwa. The person gets older as getting afraid of death. In fact, the Prophet said that there are two things corrupting human characteristics, namely loving the world and fear of death.

Explanation About Soul

Indeed, there is no soul. It means that the spirit united with the body than, it is so-called as compound / living. So when the spirit is lifted, it is called as dead. More details on the spirit with body is called as life or better known as soul. One has big or small soul because the soul has two opinions. The first opinion is from the mind of being jealousy and selfish. While the second opinion is the spirit with no jealousy, no resentment, and no sense of envy. Spirit has two colors, namely white and black. The white spirit can influence on positive actions for the body (mind) and it has been documented since in the womb. Thus, the explanation is that doing well is indeed by Allah wills.

The black spirit tends to get excited when doing something bad or make difficulty for others. Even his heart will feel happy when it sees people who do not like gets hurt. People are usually very arrogant and his heart does not want to appreciate others. When in such conditions, the important things are brain and mind. Even if that person has been written since the agreement that the he will be the prospective inhabitants of hell but then he struggles greatly to worship merely because of Allah, then Allah SWT will change the records as formerly to be a candidate for the hell into the prospective resident of heaven. Thus, the black spirit of person then is slowly going to be in white color and along by the forgiveness from Allah SWT.

Living people do not know what experience by the dead. While the dead knows what experience by living people, but it just knows and can do anything. The white spirit is in a clean condition and in white dress, while the black spirit is nude. The spirit clothes while still alive is the physical body (instinct). When died in holy- *fitrah*- condition, the spirit clothes are the *mutmainah* desire derived from the light of Muhammad who has been down to the world as *the Prophet Muhammad* (conscience). After he died, later he became the *mutmainah* desire which just wanted to live in the faithful bodies. Those are heavenly beings, eternal beings, and beings who have no boredom and creatures that have never exhausted. The realization of such creature is like you when you were in the age of 22-27 years old (virgin male) for men and for women, in the age of 17-21 years old (virgin female). The spirit getting clothes can mean as the spirit getting intercession. If worship for Allah certainly, it gets intercession but when worship because of intercession, then until whenever it will not get the intercession.

The Journey Of Led Fire

The led fire is from heaven and the nature of the led fire has three things, namely it does not burn, does not heat up and does not let. While, the nature of fire today is burning, heating, and letting, this kind of fire is from the core of earth. The journey of the led fire was first inserted into the body of Prophet Adam when he had not been sent down to earth. After a chunk of land in the earth taken by the Angel of *Azrael* on the commands of Allah and then the land was entered into fire, with little of water, and cool air from the heaven, then it was blown a spirit so, there was a living prophet who was so dashing and handsome with age of 21 years. Along the spirit was blown, Allah SWT provided a variety of knowledge which were not possessed by any demons, genies, and angels. This makes the devil to be envied to the Prophet Adam. The devil did not want to submit to Prophet Adam for maintaining its selfish nature.

Satan found only Prophet Adam who was created from clay, while Satan was created from light (the light of fire in the earth). Every time the devil continued to deny Prophet Adam and did not want to obey and respect him. Due to devil nature of arrogant, then Allah cursed the devil and later the devil would be put into hell. Nevertheless, the devils remains no sad because they had an opinion that the fire was already their place and the devils were used to it. One made the devils sad was seeing the Prophet Adam getting enjoyment. The incident was the origin of jealousy / envy.

Someone seeing his friend getting pleasure with envy, that is the devil's promptings. After the incident, the genie was frightened, so that the genie became more diligent to worship. Genie is divided into men and women while the angels are not men and not women. At the end, the genie was asked by Allah SWT and the male genie replied that he would be diligently worship because of heaven while the female genie replied that she would be diligently worship because of fear of hell. At that time, the earth condition was still in a condition which could not be called as earth because there was no up or down, no right and left, no east and west, the moon and the sun, and soil, water, fire, and wind intermingled so it could only see one lighting in quasi-silver color. When the devil was sent down to the earth, then it began to be any lumps gathered, the soil united so that there were only land and sea but the condition was no light.

The male genie worshipped increasingly diligently because of wishing to stay in heaven. Allah was wrath to the male genie who worshipped because of heaven that Allah also sent down the male genie into the sun. Since then, the male genie were given a throne in the middle of the sun and the king was named as *Ifrit*. The genie women became increasingly diligent to worship for fear of hell. Allah was wrath to the female genie who worshipped for fear of hell. The female genie were more afraid of hell than Him. Allah sent down the female genie into the month and given a throne in the middle of the month as the queen named as Balqis.

Ifrit once blocked the Prophet Muhammad while on a journey by Allah towards the *Sidrat al-Muntaha (lahw mahfuz)*. While the *Balqis* once came down to earth to tempt the Prophet Solomon AS and Devil became the mighty king in the earth. In the past, these three types of creatures were united so that they had almost the same skills equally to tempt the descendants of Prophet Adam. For the descendants of Prophet Adam who pray for Allah, the three beings cannot tempt. Therefore, brothers and sisters ,throughout our writings, it always writes to worship because of Allah (*illa mukhlisun*). Before being sent down into the seven layers of earth, the devil begged for the longevity and begged to tempt the descendants of Prophet Adam as much as possible. Allah permitted but it would not happen for His servants who worship for Allah (*illa mukhlisun*). Brothers and sisters, worship because of longevity is the first originator of devil.

The devil was condemned not for stealing or robbing, but because of his pride so that he sent down to the earth. Balqis was sent down to the moon because of worship for fear of hell while Ifrit was lowered position and sent down into the sun because of worship for heaven. Many people say that genie are also Moslem but only angels and men who can pray for Allah. If the worship because of world, it will be ease for devil to tempt. When worship for fear of hell, the female genie will be easily tempt while worship for heaven then Ifrit can arbitrarily control. Do not do anything without the knowledge and understand its origins to really understand.

The nature of fire which was led from heaven (the prophets' instinct) does not burn, meaning that in each talk, it always makes the listener to be cool. No heat means not making others angry. Not letting means to have concern for what was supposed to be and responsible with what has been delivered. Consider carefully the Islamic Shari'a namely two sentence of faith confession, prayer, alms, fasting in the holy month of Ramadan and the hajj when being able and do good to parents. The common recitation and prayer can be referred to as Islamic activities. While conducting the *sunnah* prayers, *hajad* prayers, *Dhuha* prayer, etc. depend on the obligation things - *fardhu* (Islamic Law). If the obligatory is wrong, then the whole *sunnah* will be wasted (loss condition).

The led fire came from heaven and stayed in the body of Prophet Adam. The devil is in the seven layers of earth in boasting condition with his men and became mighty king but his heart is not comfortable for revenge to the Prophet Adam. Then the devil imprisoned for 20 years and finally succeeded in ascending to heaven to see the Prophet Adam with the intention to persuade him to eat *khuldi* fruit (the banned fruit) but the Prophet Adam ignored so that the devil purpose was failed (through peacock). Then, the devil imprisoned again for 40 years with the same goal and in the end the devil managed by a snake. The devil managed to tempt the Mother of Eve with various deceits. The Prophet Adam regretted and pleaded guilty, so the Prophet Adam and mother of Eve were sent down into the earth. The Prophet Adam was sent down to the earth precisely in Hindustan while the mother Eve was sent down in the middle east. For 40 years, both were looking for each other and at the end, they met in a small mountain named as *Jabal Rahmah*.

The led fire in the Prophet Adam was never extinguished. During his life, the Prophet Adam preached to invite his people to worship only for Allah and not worship other than Him. Nine hundred years of Prophet Adam preached in hard manners and eventually died. The led fire had migrated to the baby, namely the Prophet Idris AS. While the spirit of Prophet Adam was first raised to the sky. The Prophet Idris AS was the first prophet who tamed horses. The Prophet Idris AS knew all knowledge known by the Prophet Adam. The led fire from heaven will never be extinguished but it is moved on to the prophets. When the death of the Prophet Idris AS, the led fire had gone back to God. At one time, the led fire was inserted into the baby known as *Noah AS*. The led fire could enter into the living people or the babies. An example was when the Prophet Ayub US was still alive, but the led fire could move to his son, the Prophet Yusuf.

After the led fire moved from one prophet to another prophet, it was ultimately up to mother of Siti Maryam and Prophet Isa AS when he was born. After the death of the Prophet Isa AS, the led fire was moved to the last prophet, the Prophet Muhammad SAW. The Prophet Isa AS had the knowledge from all of the previous prophets so he could receive the Holy Bible. The Great Prophet Muhammad SAW had all knowledge from all the prophets, it was no wonder that the Prophet Muhammad could tell in detail about the history of the previous prophets. Brothers and sisters, the Prophet Muhammad could know in detail the history of the previous prophets as the material for the revelation of holy Quran. That is the journey of the led fire from heaven.

Tail Bone Nerve Function

In the body anatomy, there is such thing named as coccyx. In the coccyx, there are a lot of nerves associated with balance. The nerves are directly related to the brain but through the heart. Outlining a science is the result of tail bone cooperation and the brain through the liver. When nerves in one coccyx has a good balance, the person will get the comfortable feeling and the calm mind. Maintaining balance nerves tail bone must be by maintaining the balance in any actions.

Example :

1. You are good to your father but not being good your mother, then there will be unbalanced nerves.
2. You are good to your parents but not being good to your parents-in-law, then there will be unbalanced nerves.
3. You are good to your own relatives but not being good to your wife relatives, then there will be unbalanced nerves.
4. You are good to rich people but not being good to poor people, then there will be unbalanced nerves.

If you are in good behavior and morals so, in all of the nerves the tail bone, there will be a balance and will not be problematic but it is impossible to be like that without you pass the straight path namely conducting the Islamic law because of Allah SWT. When you apply *the Islamic law* because of Allah, so you can do as we have explained by the Allah wills. The impact of unbalance coccyx nerves are:

1. Future parents can have a stroke
2. The possibility of paralysis
3. The characteristics are changed into a negative direction and getting senile
4. Proud if you have lots of money
5. Very sad if having no money
6. Easy shocked
7. The view becomes narrower in thinking
8. It seems to be very brave but in the heart, it feels fear
9. It seems to be very afraid but in the heart, it feels brave
10. Looking very happy but in the heart, it feels sad, etc.

To improve the spinal nerves, it requires a long time, but we all must try to improve morals. The heart cannot think but can be happy or sad, and can filter out something which should be delivered and that should not be delivered (to filter the toxins). The brain has a duty to define and design the strategy and govern the whole body. Improving the heart so that it can be based on its function, must worship for Allah SWT. To distinguish between the Truth and falsehood then get close to the Almighty until we are high-minded. Improving the tail bone nerves should with tangible actions so that the brain can think positively (not thinking toward something that results in the Allah's wrath).

Brothers and sisters in any country you are in, which we have described above is the real explanation (common law). While the explanation on its essence (in the Islamic faith), first to improve is the heart by applying the *Sharia Law* in a whole (the two sentence of faith confession, prayer, alms, fasting in the holy month of Ramadan, and pilgrimage when being able because of Allah SWT as well as being good the parents and parents in-laws). If the heart has faith, it will run its function well which is to filter the words and actions and morals. If so, surely the way of brain thinking will not likely deviate everywhere so it automatically the coccyx along with its nerves will always be balanced and will not likely be affected by any diseases which we have mentioned above.

Humans can take lessons if they have *faith*. Humans can be *faith* if worshipping for Allah. While most humans worship for other than Allah (to indulge one's own desires). Indeed, the humans are in loss condition. Thus, when the brain is always thinking toward something that results in the Allah's wrath. Someone who fails to the devil and genie temptation is not because the devils and genie are clever but it is because of the human stupidity. From this long-writing, we provide this merely not jst as knowledge but as the forerunner of knowledge as the basic materials for researches. Only the great nations who want to think and will be interested. Islam cannot be outdated and there is no expiration. The world is currently in drowning conditions, namely drowning in happiness, drowning in distress, drowning in a sea of arrogance and drowning in anger as well as that there are many complaints which cannot accept the provisions of Allah SWT. Let us get back on the straight paths, namely the paths brought by the Prophet Muhammad SAW.

www.ingramcontent.com/pod-product-compliance
Lightning Source LLC
Chambersburg PA
CBHW051439280526
45785CB00003B/1354